COMPLEX AND TRAUMATIC LOSS

Also Available

Normal Family Processes:
Growing Diversity and Complexity, Fourth Edition
Edited by Froma Walsh

Spiritual Resources in Family Therapy, Second Edition
Edited by Froma Walsh

Strengthening Family Resilience, Third Edition
Froma Walsh

Complex and Traumatic Loss

Fostering Healing and Resilience

Froma Walsh

gp

THE GUILFORD PRESS
New York   London

Copyright © 2023 The Guilford Press
A Division of Guilford Publications, Inc.
370 Seventh Avenue, Suite 1200, New York, NY 10001
www.guilford.com

Printed in the United States of America

This book is printed on acid-free paper.

Last digit is print number: 9   8   7   6   5   4   3   2   1

Library of Congress Cataloging-in-Publication data is available from the publisher.

ISBN 978-1-4625-5302-0 (paperback)

ISBN 978-1-4625-5255-9 (cloth)

About the Author

Froma Walsh, MSW, PhD, is the Mose and Sylvia Firestone Professor Emerita in the Crown Family School of Social Work, Policy, and Practice and the Department of Psychiatry, Pritzker School of Medicine, University of Chicago. She is also Co-Founder and Co-Director of the Chicago Center for Family Health. Dr. Walsh is an internationally respected clinical scholar and a foremost authority on family resilience. Integrating developmental, relational, sociocultural, and spiritual perspectives, her resilience-oriented systemic approach with individuals, couples, and families fosters healing and positive adaptation. She is past editor of the *Journal of Marital and Family Therapy* and past president of the American Family Therapy Academy. Dr. Walsh is the recipient of many honors for distinguished contributions to theory, research, and practice, including the Presidential Citation from the American Psychological Association and awards from the American Family Therapy Academy, the American Association for Marriage and Family Therapy, the American Orthopsychiatric Association, and the Society for Pastoral Counseling Research. She is a frequent speaker and consultant internationally, and her books have been translated into many languages.

Preface

Of all life experiences, death and loss pose the most painful challenges in adaptation, with reverberations in all relationships and life pursuits. This book, designed for mental health, healthcare, community service, and pastoral professionals, provides a research-informed, resilience-oriented systemic framework to guide therapeutic practice with individuals, couples, and families in grieving, healing, and positive adaptation with complex and traumatic loss.

While loss and grief are universal human experiences, every experience is unique and dependent on many variables, such as the timing, circumstances, and significance of the death. This volume highlights the most current advances in our knowledge and understanding of a range of complicated and traumatic loss situations. Research has made clear that mourning and adaptational processes are varied, lengthy, and complex: there is no right way to grieve and no fixed sequence of stages to a complete resolution. Therefore, rather than presenting a treatment manual or "one-size-fits-all" set of techniques, this text provides practice principles to guide therapy, addressing both common and unique challenges and recovery pathways in varied loss situations; individual, couple, and family impact; and sociocultural contexts.

The most current science on human resilience in response to trauma (Masten & Motti-Stefanidi, 2020) has shifted from an individual focus to a broad systemic perspective, recognizing the mutual interactions of individual, family, and larger social influences that increase risk of dysfunction or support healing and positive adaptation. This volume is distinct in the current professional literature on loss and grief in presenting a resilience-oriented, systemic approach. Textbooks for training and practice with loss and grief focus predominantly on individual, symptom-focused treatments, and the few that focus on resilience and positive growth give scant attention to influences in family and social contexts. This volume expands the lens to understand and address the powerful impact of death and loss in the family relational system, affecting all members and their relationships, family functioning, and hopes and dreams for all that might have been. A significant loss leaves a hole in the heart of the family.

To reflect today's diverse societies, this approach is broadly inclusive of the varied and complex relational patterns, values, and life course in intimate bonds, childrearing, and extended kin and social networks. In this volume, gender-inclusive singular pronouns *they/them/their* are used throughout. The relational terms *spouse/partner/parent/child* are used unless gender-specific issues are relevant in particular situations or case examples. We also attend to workplace, healthcare, and larger systems stresses and inequities that heighten the risks of traumatic death and complications in grieving and adaptation.

This practice approach builds on core principles and methods of strength-based, collaborative, systemic therapies in the field of family therapy. A resilience-oriented approach attends to the experience of loss and deep suffering, the challenges posed for adaptation, and the human capacity for resilience, helping those struggling to heal and forge pathways forward to thrive. It addresses the grief, contextualizes distress, strengthens relevant couple and family processes, and supports the bereaved in mobilizing vital social, economic, cultural, and spiritual resources. When working primarily with individuals, therapists can address these influences through coaching methods or may flexibly combine couple or family sessions, as well as group formats.

With this approach, therapists can facilitate both individual and relational healing and resilience. For instance, while some studies report that the death of a child heightens the risk for divorce, other studies find that couples' relationships are often strengthened when they provide mutual support through their painful experience. With the loss of a family breadwinner or primary caregiver, help beyond griefwork can facilitate functional role realignment. The worst of times can bring out the best in individuals and deepen their bonds. Many find meaning through their struggles to take more purposeful directions in their lives. We can assist in these transformations.

Because stories can illuminate the experience of complicated loss to inform our therapeutic response, readers will find many vignettes of real-life situations and clinical case examples throughout the volume. (To protect confidentiality, each is carefully disguised or is a composite of cases and therapeutic work.) I believe clinicians have much to learn from stories of ordinary people, revealing both their suffering and their extraordinary strengths in surmounting shattering losses.

THE AUDIENCE FOR THIS BOOK

This volume is designed for a broad professional readership in training and therapeutic practice across disciplines and settings. This includes psychologists, counselors, social workers, marriage and family therapists, and psychiatrists; physicians, nurses, and hospice workers; humanitarian aid workers; and pastoral counselors, chaplains, and clergy. The volume also serves well as a basic text for college and graduate courses addressing death, dying, and bereavement in the social sciences; human development; and child and family studies.

Reflecting a resilience-based systemic practice approach, the term *therapist* is used broadly, to be inclusive of counselors and clinicians across disciplines who work with clients (patients) in therapeutic practice. Loss and grief are viewed not as disorders to treat, but as normal human suffering, with therapeutic efforts aimed to support and strengthen our clients' inherent potential for healing and resilience.

Our culture minimizes the impact of loss and grief, urging rapid closure. In faulty notions of resilience, the bereaved are offered cheery advice to "be strong" and "bounce back." For many, help seeking is stigmatized and shame laden. Traditional gender-based socialization still constrains many men from expressing grief and emotionally supporting loved ones.

Whether in general practice or specialty services, most practitioners will be called upon to address tragic losses and complicated bereavement, both in the aftermath of loss and, in some cases, long after a death. Yet, insufficient attention to loss in professional training across disciplines, except for grief specialists, leaves most therapists ill equipped to understand and address loss-related concerns when they arise. Some seek help directly for their grief; others may present somatic, behavioral, relational, or child-focused problems that reverberate from the loss, when grief was unaddressed or unsupported. Some only seek help years later, when submerged pain from past loss surfaces in other life problems and relationships, often not initially noting the connection.

In these turbulent times, we will need to help those who have lost loved ones in pandemic-related deaths and others bereaved in the growing numbers of deaths in gun violence, addiction, and suicide. Families and communities will need help in grieving and rebuilding lives after collective losses in climate-related disasters, war, refugee uprooting, and mass shootings. Greater attention is also needed to the bereaved in underserved low-income, racial/ethnic, and sexual minority communities that suffer higher risk of mortality and fewer healthcare and therapeutic resources. To meet these urgent demands, greater attention to the impact of loss is needed in all clinical training and practices to foster healing and resilience.

EVOLUTION OF THEORY, RESEARCH, AND PRACTICE IN MY WORK

The importance of a resilience-oriented systemic approach to address loss and grief has been a central clinical focus in my scholarly publications, teaching, therapy practice, and community consultations throughout my career.

In the early development of family systems theory, Murray Bowen and others first described the ripple effects of complicated mourning in couple and family relationships and in family functioning. Monica McGoldrick and I, in separate clinical studies in New Jersey and Chicago, respectively, discussed our findings and began a rich collaboration aiming to advance systemic understandings and interventions with loss. In 1988 we organized an international conference on loss at Ballymaloe, Ireland, inviting international colleagues engaged in family systems research and practice. This led to our coedited book, *Living Beyond Loss: Death in the Family* (Walsh & McGoldrick, 1991, 2004), which became a landmark text in the clinical literature. Since then, systems-based articles have remained scattered in journals and multitopic volumes (e.g., Nadeau, 2008; Rosenblatt; 2013; Walsh, 2019; Walsh & McGoldrick, 2013), unintegrated in practice by most clinicians. Colleagues have urged me to meet the need for a new textbook for practitioners.

Over recent decades, my conceptual framework and practice approach with loss have been enriched by emerging research in the field and by my ongoing clinical teaching and consultation experience. At the University of Chicago, I taught a large seminar for many years on Loss, Recovery, and Resilience for students in social work, psychology, human development, and pastoral counseling. Over 30 years, as co-director of the university-affiliated advanced training institute, the Chicago Center for Family Health, I have offered seminars and supervision on working with bereaved families. I have also provided training and consultation nationally and internationally in a resilience-oriented approach for counselors working in collective trauma situations (such as the aftermath of Hurricane Katrina; United Nations Relief and Works Agency services in Gaza and the West Bank; refugees from Bosnia and Kosovo; and gang prevention/youth development efforts in Los Angeles).

The practice approach presented here is grounded in the family resilience framework I developed over four decades, informed by the research literature, my own studies, and extensive experience in training professionals and in therapeutic practice. Regrettably, systems-oriented studies on loss remain few to date. I hope this volume will encourage more research efforts to examine the family-wide implications of a tragic death, family and social processes that support adaptation over time, and the larger systemic and sociocultural variables in risk and resilience. Mixed-methods research is essential, with qualitative studies to further illuminate meaning-making processes and other subjectivities in the experience of loss. Because research funding and clinical studies have had a skewed focus on risk and dysfunction, it is crucial to give more attention to family strengths and social resources that support healing and resilience.

STRUCTURE AND CONTENTS OF THE BOOK

Chapters throughout this volume address many difficult situations of complicated and traumatic loss, the challenges and struggles of the bereaved, and practice principles to support healing grief processes and the human capacity for resilience.

The book is organized into three sections. *Part I* provides an overview of a resilience-oriented systemic practice approach with painful losses and adaptational challenges, considering individual, couples, family, and larger sociocultural and spiritual influences. Chapter 1 summarizes research advances in understanding grief and adaptation to loss and expands the predominant individual, dyadic focus of treatment to a systems perspective, attending to the reverberations of loss in couple and family processes that can hinder or support positive adaptation. Chapter 2 describes core principles in a resilience-oriented practice approach with loss and applies my family resilience framework, which guides discussion throughout the volume to foster individual and relational healing and resilience. Chapter 3 examines the intertwined influence of cultural beliefs and multigenerational norms and addresses common constraints of gender-based socialization. It attends to the significance of spiritual beliefs in death, dying, and loss; the mystery of afterlife; and existential concerns, offering a guide to explore their role in suffering and potential resources in healing and resilience.

In *Part II*, Chapters 4–6 address the common challenges patients and their loved ones face in approaching death and dying, and in the wake of loss for the bereaved. Chapter 4 attends to anticipated loss with terminal illness and to anguishing end-of-life concerns. Chapter 5 describes family adaptational challenges in bereavement to guide clinicians in facilitating individual and shared processes that support grieving and moving forward in life. Practice principles and guidelines are offered to work effectively with individuals, couples, and families in individual and conjoint sessions. Chapter 6 provides a family developmental perspective and practice guidelines with the death of a spouse, parent, child, sibling, grandparent, or grandchild at different life phases and varied family forms.

In *Part III*, Chapters 7–13 provide crucial information to understand traumatic loss situations and practice principles in working sensitively to address complex emotional and practical challenges for healing and resilience. Chapter 7 first discusses situations of ambiguous loss, as in the unknown fate of a missing loved one or in progressive cognitive impairment with dementias. It then addresses disenfranchised grief, when a significant loss is socially unacknowledged, minimized, or stigmatized, as in pregnancy and perinatal losses; deaths in significant nonfamily bonds; or with a hidden relationship or cause of death. Chapter 8 deals with the complicated loss of a cherished companion animal: helping children, adults, and families when their grief is trivialized; with traumatic loss situations; and with decisions to euthanize a pet. Chapter 9 addresses the devastating impact of losses in violent and traumatic circumstances, including a fatal accident, homicide, relational abuse, alcohol- or drug-related death, and suicide. Chapter 10 attends to losses complicated by relational dynamics in highly conflicted, abusive, or estranged relationships and addresses current distress reverberating from past traumatic losses and transgenerational transmission. Chapter 11 addresses the complex losses and adaptational challenges for individuals, families, and communities impacted by collective trauma, including major disasters; war and conflict-regions; refugee experience; gun violence; and mass killings. Principles in resilience-oriented, multilevel systemic intervention are described.

Finally, Chapter 12 explores the shared human experience of loss, examining therapists' own professional, personal, and familial influences and ways they may constrain or can enrich our therapeutic work. The emotional intensity of a tragic loss situation and the grief responses of the bereaved require therapist awareness of the interface issues that contribute to compassion fatigue. To encourage readers' own explorations, my reflections and colleagues' brief vignettes relate our personal experiences, multigenerational family legacies, and how they can inspire meaningful professional pursuits.

The loss of a loved one is one of the most intensely painful experiences any human being can suffer. Rippling in effect through relational systems, it can shatter couple and family bonds, with long-term ramifications. It is also challenging for therapists to witness and address, as death is not a problem that can be solved—we cannot bring back the deceased. Our compassion and support in people's potential to heal and adapt out of tragedy can encourage their best efforts to find meaning, reorient hope, and go forward to live and love fully.

Acknowledgments

I want to thank the dedicated staff at The Guilford Press for their professionalism and collaborative spirit in the production of this new volume. I especially appreciate the superb oversight of Senior Production Editor Jeannie Tang, the creative responsiveness of Art Director Paul Gordon, the thoughtful efforts of Senior Copy Manager Katherine Lieber, and the eagle eye of Associate Editor Jane Keislar. I am most grateful for the valuable feedback provided by Senior Editor Jim Nageotte, who has been my trusted "North Star," guiding my path throughout this project.

Writing this book has been a labor of love. Yet the overwhelming losses and upheaval wrought by the lengthy pandemic made me question, at times, whether it was all too much to try to address a wide range of complicated and traumatic loss situations, the profound distress of loved ones, and the ripple effects in their lives and relational networks over time and across generations. In a post-pandemic context, would anyone even buy and read a book about death and loss? It was a lonely project. When people asked me what my new book was about, in hearing the words "death" and "loss" most said nothing, changed the subject, and never asked again about the book or expressed any interest. Yet, this is why I felt the need to write this book. Our society avoids the topic of death, presses the bereaved to "bounce back," and pathologizes "prolonged grief." Some who suppress their pain come for help, often years later, presenting other problems reverberating from past loss. My hope is that this book can reach helping professionals across disciplines and specialties, offering a guide to understand and address the suffering, adaptational challenges, and systemic influences with tragic losses and to support the human potential for healing and resilience.

I am grateful to my colleagues, friends, and family members who have expanded and deepened my understanding of death, dying, and bereavement. First and foremost was my early collaboration with Monica McGoldrick, building on the pioneering studies in the bereavement and family systems fields, and sharing insights from our separate research and practice experiences and those of our colleagues. This new volume is informed by the systemic framework we developed to understand the impact of significant losses in family systems. Over the past three decades, my work has been greatly enriched by my experiences in teaching, research, supervision, and stimulating exchanges with faculty colleagues and students at the Chicago Center for Family Health and in the Crown Family School (formerly SSA) at the University of Chicago. I want to thank my longtime clinical colleagues, William Borden and Stanley McCracken, for our wide-ranging, ongoing conversations about therapy, life, and loss. I look forward to future contacts and collaborations with colleagues globally to advance systemic approaches in both research and practice.

I have learned the most from the individuals, couples, and families I've been privileged to work with at times of death, dying, and bereavement. They have taught me about dignity, humanity, and generosity in the face of suffering, struggle, and limits of control. Even more, they have demonstrated the possibilities for personal and relational healing and transformation through the worst of times, forged with courage, compassion, and resourcefulness.

My family and the kinship of close friends have been a wellspring for meaningful connection, joy, and resilience in my life. I hold in precious remembrance those who have been there for me in times of my own life-threatening crises and painful losses; they taught me the vital importance of relational support. My husband, John Rolland, has been my personal and professional mainstay and has informed my work in his integrative approach with couples and families facing terminal illness. I admire my daughter, Claire Whitney, for her compassionate commitment to her career in international humanitarian work, building capacities for mental health and psychosocial support to foster recovery and resilience in global settings of overwhelming crisis and loss. Above all, I am grateful to my parents for raising me with loving care despite their own life struggles and unspeakable losses. Their memory is an abiding blessing.

Contents

PART I

Overview

CHAPTER 1

Facing Death and Loss

The Human Predicament

> In coming to accept death, we can more fully embrace life.
> —VIKTOR FRANKL, *Man's Search for Meaning*

Of all human experiences, death and loss pose the most painful and far-reaching challenges for loved ones. Unbearable, shattering, devastating, unspeakable are words commonly used to capture the impact of a tragic loss. Bereavement theory, research, and practice have focused primarily on individual grief after the loss of a significant dyadic bond. Yet the impact of a death ripples through entire relational networks, touching many lives with immediate and long-term ramifications. Couple and family bonds can be broken; hopes and dreams may be shattered. The submerged pain of overwhelming loss may surface years later in problematic behavior, relationships, or life pursuits, which bring people to therapy.

This book expands our lens to address grief and adaptation to loss in light of complex systemic processes in situations of complicated and traumatic loss. Applying a resilience-oriented framework, the approach presented here attends both to the experience of deep suffering and to the human capacity for adaptation and positive growth. With this approach, practitioners working with individuals, couples, families, and other relational systems can address risk factors for maladaptation and can facilitate relational processes and supportive resources to heal from grief and to live and love fully in the wake of loss.

OVERCOMING AVERSION TO ATTENDING TO DEATH AND LOSS

Mental health professionals work with many situations of extreme suffering, ranging from serious health and mental health conditions to addictions, violence, and sexual abuse; we treat widespread trauma effects in the ravages of war, community disasters, and global pandemics. Yet many practitioners are uneasy in approaching death and loss. Our own anxieties are aroused because we must all experience their impact. There is no safe boundary between professionals and our patients/clients: we, the helpers, are all vulnerable, facing the inevitability of our own mortality and the devastating loss of loved ones and others important in our lives.

Irving Yalom (2009) observed that living with awareness of death is like trying to stare directly at the sun—we can glance, but we quickly look away. We all have difficulty facing our anxiety. Highway traffic slows down to witness a crash site—then speeds up again; it could have been us. For some, the fear can lead to unhealthy rumination; for others, it can go underground, surfacing later and in other relationships. Some seek escape in overwork or affairs, in alcohol or drugs. Others defy (or invite) death in risk-taking behavior. Yet, as Yalom contends, we cannot live or love fully if we are frozen in fear or denial. Rather, by facing it and grasping our human condition, we can savor the preciousness of each moment and more fully live and gain compassion for ourselves and for all others.

DEATH AND LOSS IN SOCIOHISTORICAL CONTEXT

Families over the ages have had to cope with the precariousness of life and disruptions wrought by death. Before modern medicine, death frequently struck young and old alike—as tragically, it continues to do in marginalized and underresourced communities. Even when commonplace, each death is a profound loss for loved ones. Until 20th-century medical advances, the life expectancy in North America was just 47 years—an age now considered midlife. Parental death often disrupted family units, shifting members into varied and complex kinship networks. Before the advent of hospital and institutional care, people died at home, where all family members, including children, were involved in preparing for death. Modern technological society fostered the avoidance of grief processes as Western medicine, hospitals, and nursing homes removed the frail and dying from everyday life and community supports. Geographical distances and pressured work schedules in modern life increasingly hindered direct contact of family members at times of death and dying.

Across cultures and faiths worldwide, mourning beliefs and practices have facilitated both the integration of death and the transformation of survivors, who must carry on with life (see Chapter 3). Most traditions hold a worldview and rituals that facilitate acceptance of the inescapable fact of death, including it in the rhythm of life, the passage to a spiritual realm, and an abiding faith in a higher power. Most approach loss as an occasion for family and community cohesion and mutual support.

The dominant Anglo-American culture, in contrast, has fostered avoidance in facing death and has encouraged the bereaved to minimize the profound impact of loss (Becker, 1973). Western medicine has tended to view death as a failure of treatment. Workplace systems expect a rapid return to job responsibilities, and few offer paid bereavement leave. Our ethos of "the rugged individual" urges the bereaved to quickly gain "closure," "get over it," and move on with life. A dichotomous view prevails in masculine images: "staying strong versus falling apart." Reflecting this cultural aversion, the training and practice of mental and behavioral health professionals have been slow to recognize and address loss-related issues.

Yet, there has been a growing recognition of the importance of attending to anticipated loss with life-threatening conditions and to care for the dying and the bereaved (see Chapter 4). Developments in palliative and hospice care ease suffering and provide support and comfort to patients and families facing end-of-life challenges. Still, sudden, preventable, and untimely deaths are all too common in underresourced, racial/ethnic communities and other marginalized groups.

The internet and social media have expanded attention to widespread traumatic losses in catastrophic events worldwide, from major disasters to war and mass killings (see Chapter 11). We have been navigating perilous times through the COVID-19 pandemic, with heightened awareness of the precariousness of life and death and multiple losses in our volatile and uncertain global environment. The tragedy for each bereaved family can be obscured by statistics, particularly when others are eager to move on. The need is all the more urgent for therapists to attend to the bereaved and to support their positive adaptation going forward.

Amid the social, economic, and political upheavals of our times, many families are dealing with multiple losses, disruptions, and uncertainties. This volume focuses on loss through death; yet, the adaptational challenges and intervention approach described have broader applicability to other disruptive life experiences involving loss, such as migration, unemployment, illness/disability, family separation, divorce, foster care, and adoption (Harris, 2020). By attending to their grief and life disruptions and in strengthening their resilience, we can help those affected to deepen vital bonds and forge new strengths.

LOSS IN COUPLES, FAMILIES, AND OTHER RELATIONAL SYSTEMS

Our understanding of loss and our clinical approaches with those in distress must be attuned to our clients' relational lives and their social contexts. Couples and families today are increasingly diverse and complex, each weaving a web of intimate bonds and kinship ties within and across households and geographic locations and over an expanded life course (Walsh, 2012). Demographic trends reveal growing cultural diversity; varied family structures, role relations, gender identity, and sexual orientation, as well as socioeconomic and racial disparities in resources and life chances.

A broad view of family and other significant bonds is crucial to understand the meaning and significance of losses in immediate and extended relationships. Families may involve multigenerational and social networks, and they may be defined by blood, legal, and/or historical ties; by formal and informal kinship bonds; by residential patterns within and across households; and by past and/or future commitments. Bonds with cherished companion animals can bring profound grief with their loss (see Chapter 8). Many persons consider their closest friends or interpersonal networks as their "kindred spirits" or chosen families, as is common in lesbian, gay, bisexual, transgender, queer, and other gender or sexual variant (LGBTQI+) communities. The impact of loss can also reverberate throughout closely knit workplace, healthcare, and educational networks, faith congregations, and communities. Systemic responses in each situation can facilitate individual, relational, and group healing and resilience.

UNDERSTANDING LOSS IN SYSTEMIC PERSPECTIVE

Attention to bereavement in clinical theory, research, and practice has focused primarily on individual grief reactions to the loss of a significant dyadic bond. In the family, a parental death for a child is also a spousal loss for a surviving parent and the loss of a child for grandparents. Individual members who are not symptomatic or seeking help are often presumed not to need attention. Yet, the impact of a significant loss ripples across the relational field, touching all others and their bonds, even years later, and affecting those who may not have even known the deceased.

In my clinical experience, a husband may send his intensely grieving wife for counseling after the death of their child, while distancing from her sorrow and his own, not knowing how to be helpful or checking his own grief to keep strong and function on his job. The wife, in contrast to her empathic therapist, may feel abandoned by her spouse, with mutual withdrawal and alienation. In another situation, a wife, overwhelmed emotionally by the sudden death of her beloved father, turns on her husband, raging at his every fault; she abruptly leaves him and moves away, leaving their confused and abandoned children in the wake. Two years later, he seeks therapy, still trying to make sense of the divorce and his personal faults, wanting to help his kids who are hurting and hesitant to trust a new intimate relationship.

Attachment theory has offered an understanding of the roots of grief in early-life dyadic bonds with a primary caregiver (Bowlby, 1982). Insecure early attachments can influence not only painful difficulties with the loss of that bond, but also problematic reactions to bereavement in other relationships in life, including prolonged or blocked grief, anxiety, and depression (Rubin, Malkinson, & Witzum, 2012). Byng-Hall (2004) expanded Bowlby's dyadic perspective to the relational system, stressing the importance of a secure family base and showing how complex dynamics affect family loss processes across the generations (see Chapter 10).

A systems orientation attends to the interactional processes and mutual influences throughout the relational network. Loss is a powerful nodal experience that shakes the foundation of family life. Individual distress stems not only from grief, but also from the realignment of the family structure and emotional field, affecting marital, sibling, and intergenerational relationships. Murray Bowen (1978) and others observed how death or threatened loss can disrupt a family's functional equilibrium. The intensity of the reaction is influenced by the significance of the lost member, by the circumstances of the death, and by relational dynamics and family functioning at the time of the loss, as will be addressed in the chapters throughout this volume.

Family cohesion can be shattered with a traumatic loss, each member reacting in their own ways and without relational support (see Chapter 9). One child may be withdrawn, depressed, or anxious, while another sibling may externalize distress in problematic behavior and yet another may seem to be unaffected or will act cheerfully to support an overwhelmed parent (see Chapter 6). Parents may deflect their grief by focusing on a symptomatic child, who is brought in for individual therapy, when the whole family is suffering and is needing help.

Many months after the mother's death to cancer, Zoe, 19, away at college, was crying uncontrollably and unable to study; individual grief counseling was unhelpful. At home, her brother, Greg, age 12, was isolated in his room, immersed in video games. Her sister Denise, 16, kept

cheerfully attentive to their widowed father, who was preoccupied with
his demanding job.

    The father and daughters came for a family consultation session with
me. (The son had refused to come.) Denise sat close to the father; Zoe sat
across the room, near the door. I began by offering my condolences for
their loss and asked them how our session might be helpful. The father
looked over at Zoe, who replied, "I can't stop crying." I asked, "Have
you all shared your tears with each other?" Zoe responded, "I feel like I
have all the tears for everyone. My brother's checked out. My sister's acting like the little mother, taking care of our father—and Dad [turning to
him]: You act like you don't even care that Mom died!" I asked, "Would
it help if your dad could share his tears?" She nodded vigorously, "Yes,
yes!" As Denise reached out to pat her father's arm, I asked her thoughts.
"I worry that he loved my mother so much, he could fall apart or just
disappear and we would lose him, too. So, I try to keep his spirits up."
Turning to their father, I asked how this terrible loss has been for him.
He replied, "It's all too much to bear, so I try to keep strong for my kids
and just keep functioning." Acknowledging the pain and concerns of
each of them, and noting the son's absence, I observed how hard it is to
grieve such a huge loss alone and how beneficial their mutual support
could be in their healing process. The father nodded, adding, "I didn't
realize how much we all need each other to get through this—and how
they need me to help them."

Beyond the grief reactions of the closest members, emotional shock
waves can reverberate throughout the relational network, immediately or
long after a death. Unbearable losses can fuel strong reactions in other relationships—from marital conflict, distancing, and divorce to precipitous
replacement or extramarital affairs (Paul & Paul, 1986). In our separate
early research and clinical practice, Monica McGoldrick and I observed
serious complications of past traumatic losses throughout the family system and across generations (McGoldrick & Walsh, 1983; Walsh, 1983;
Walsh & McGoldrick, 1991, 2004; see Chapter 10).

    How the family handles the loss situation has far-reaching effects, as
I have seen in my practice over the years.

Hope, a divorced woman in her 50s, came for individual therapy at the
urging of her adult children, who complained, "You've got to stop over-
mothering us—we're grown adults with children of our own!" While
generally in good health, Hope suffered for many years with fibromyalgia.

    In the first session, Hope said she couldn't help worrying—she
didn't know how to be a mother of adult children, since she had lost

her own mother to cancer when she was 7. As we explored that loss, she recalled feeling abandoned in the months before the death, as her father hovered over her mother and tried to shelter her from child care burdens. She recalled the last night, when relatives gathered behind closed doors in the parents' bedroom, where her mother lay dying. Hope dressed her younger brother and herself in their Sunday best, and they sat holding hands, waiting to be called in to say their good-byes, but no one came for them. In the chaotic days that followed, they weren't taken to the funeral, with well-intentioned relatives believing it would be too upsetting for them. As their father was too overwhelmed in his grief to care for them, two aunts each took in a sibling, separating them from mutual support, with anxious uncertainty when or if they would return home to their father.

On their return several weeks later, the father, isolated in his unbearable grief, drank heavily and came into her bed at night, sexually abusing her. Her secret torment continued until he remarried a year later. Listening with compassion to her story, I noted that Hope showed no anger in relating this abuse—the first time she had ever revealed it to anyone. She said she never blamed her father because she felt so sorry for his deep sadness and loneliness; it comforted him and eased her fear of losing her only surviving parent.

Years later, Hope married a man who was a heavy drinker. She endured his physical abuse for many years to keep her family intact for her children until they were grown. I asked about her brother. She said their close bond remained her lifeline over the years—they checked in with each other daily. It was only at that point in our sessions that she broke down sobbing, revealing that Jim had died a year ago in the crash of a small plane.

Legacies of loss find expression in far-ranging patterns of interaction and mutual influence among the survivors and across the generations. Therefore, it's important for therapists to assess the relational system and the family dynamics surrounding loss to understand the meaning and context of presenting difficulties. As in this case, some families fall apart after an unbearable loss, with surviving partners/parents unable to provide needed comfort, reassurance, and security in the aftermath. Anxieties with secondary losses of separation, unclear communication, and future uncertainty increase suffering. Sibling bonds can be vital lifelines through loss and disruption and for years to come. The recent tragic death of Hope's brother was a devastating loss of her primary bond and reactivated her childhood trauma, with reverberations in her relationships with her adult children. The biopsychosocial interconnections of painful loss also emerged in a flare-up of her fibromyalgia.

A systemic approach is a conceptual orientation to practice, whether working with individuals, couples, families, or communities. In addressing loss from a systemic perspective, we attend not only to individual grief but also to family processes and larger contextual influences that constrain or facilitate healing and resilience, as will be considered in the chapters that follow. The complex meanings of a particular loss event and individual responses to it are shaped by family belief systems and significant life experiences. A loss may also modify the family structure, requiring reorganization of roles and other relationships. A death in the family system involves multiple losses and reconfigurations in numerous relationships, in role functioning, and in the family unit:

- Loss of the person
- Loss of each member's unique bond
- Loss of functional roles
- Loss of the intact family unit
- Loss of hopes and dreams for all that might have been

The impact of loss is greater the more central the role the deceased had, such as primary breadwinner, caregiver, or matriarch. Loss of the love of one's life or an only child leaves a particular void. Grief in highly conflicted or estranged relationships may be unexpectedly strong and often more painful because it is too late to repair bonds. Widespread catastrophic events, such as disasters, epidemics, or war or political oppression, may involve multiple losses and displacement in kin and social networks, homes and communities, schools, jobs, and income security.

When significant losses have been unattended, symptoms are more likely to appear in a child, or spousal conflict may erupt, without connecting such reactions to the loss. Therefore, to better understand the meaning of symptoms and to facilitate healing, it is important to assess the relational configuration, the significance of painful losses, and the family's transactional processes surrounding the loss.

BEREAVEMENT IN SOCIAL AND DEVELOPMENTAL CONTEXTS

The meanings and ramifications of loss vary depending on the intersection of multiple variables, including the nature and circumstances of a death, the state of relationships, family functioning, sociocultural influences, and the phase of individual and family life-cycle passage at the time of loss, as will be addressed in the chapters that follow.

An ecosystemic orientation (Bateson, 1979) informs our work with the dying and bereaved. We attend to interconnected biopsychosocial influences in adaptation to loss, with expanded attention to the social context. It may be important to address barriers in healthcare, financial, and other resources that constrain adaptation and to mobilize practical and emotional supports in extended kin and social networks, communities, educational and work settings, and other larger systems. Socioeconomic inequities and marginalization involving poverty, racism, sexism, hetero-sexism, and other forms of discrimination render disadvantaged groups at higher risk for fatal conditions, traumatic losses, and complications in adaptation (McDowell, Knudson-Martin, & Bermudez, 2019).

Like the social context, the temporal context holds a matrix of mean-ings, influencing present and future adaptations with loss. From a develop-mental systems perspective, death and loss are not simply discrete events. They involve many interwoven processes connecting the deceased and sur-vivors and significant others over time—from the threat and approach of death, through the immediate disruption and aftermath for the bereaved, and on to long-term implications in life strivings and other relationships. The unbearable heaviness of remembering leads some to disconnect from themselves, their past, their loved ones, and new attachments. In clinical practice, clients may present individual or relational problems that stem from or reactivate past loss experiences, often out of their awareness of connection.

A family life-cycle perspective attends to the mutual influences within and across generations as they respond to loss and move forward over time (see Chapters 6 and 10). Current difficulties may be exacerbated by a pileup of stressors or previous adverse experiences. We consider past, present, and future connections, not in deterministic causal assumptions, but rather in exploring their possible relevance. Each loss ties in with all other losses and yet is unique in its meaning. The ability to accept and integrate loss as a natural and inevitable milestone in the life cycle is at the heart of healthy processes in human systems. Although loss is painful and disruptive, sharing grief with kin and community facilitates healing and the ability to reengage fully with life.

ADVANCES IN UNDERSTANDING
GRIEF AND ADAPTATION TO LOSS

Contemporary approaches to bereavement, grounded in extensive research, have advanced from earlier griefwork models, which were heavily influ-enced by Anglo-American cultural norms and psychoanalytic theory. Based on assumptions about normal versus abnormal grief, they purported a single, universal standard of normal grief, with other responses viewed as pathological. Clinical approaches have evolved from a simple "one-size-fits-all" griefwork model to appreciate the varied and complex mourning processes in family, social, and developmental contexts. Current best practices emphasize the following:

1. There are many varied ways to grieve and adapt to loss. There is no single "right" or "best" way for healthy bereavement. Epidemiological and cross-cultural studies have documented a wide variation in the timing, expression, and intensity of individual grief responses (Wortman & Silver, 2001). Sociocultural standards, religious teachings, family traditions, and personal differences influence a wide range of mourning approaches.

2. Grief processes do not follow an orderly progression or stage sequence, as proposed by Kübler-Ross and Kessler (2005). Common reactions of shock and disbelief, anger, bargaining, sorrow, and acceptance are better seen as facets of grief, which ebb and flow over time and can resurface with unexpected intensity. Sorrow and yearning for all that was lost are most common. Yet, popularized notions of passage through stages of grief have persisted in faulty linear expectations of progress and completion that too often compound the pain of loss (Stroebe, Schut, & Boerner, 2017).

3. Adaptation to loss does not mean resolution, as in some complete "once-and-for-all" getting over it. Significant losses may never be fully resolved, and grief may resurface years later or persist over a lifetime. Therefore, I prefer not to use the term unresolved loss to refer to troubling or unaddressed issues that may bring people to therapy. Mourning and recovery are gradual, fluid processes, usually lessening in intensity over the months and years following a loss. Yet various facets of grief are commonly aroused, particularly at anniversaries, birthdays, and milestones.

4. Adaptive coping involves a dynamic oscillation of attention between loss and restoration. In dual processes, the focus of the bereaved alternates: at times on grief and at other times on emerging life challenges (Stroebe & Schut, 2010). Beyond brief grief-focused counseling in early bereavement, therapeutic attention may be needed to address the practical, emotional, and relational challenges for survivors in reorienting their lives. Some may not seek therapy until many months after a death, when the immediate crush of responsibilities subsides and social support wanes.

5. Continuing bonds: Transformation of bonds. Death ends a life but not relationships. Past grief theory emphasized the importance of "letting go" and detachment from the deceased. Healthy mourning processes are now seen as a transformation of emotional connection from physical presence to continuing bonds (Klass, Silverman, & Nickman, 2014; Walsh & McGoldrick, 2004). These bonds are sustained through spiritual connections, memories, stories, photos, deeds, other relationships, and legacies passed on to future generations.

6. Grief is a healing process over time: We don't get over it; we move forward through it. We often speak of the recovery process as a journey, yet it is not a journey anyone chooses, and it does not have a final destination. The path forward has many twists and turns, with few guideposts along the way. Clinicians do well to slow down pressure by clients and well-intentioned others for rushed and rapid "closure" of painful emotions. Although loss is disruptive, we heal and grow stronger by going through it, not by getting over it.

7. We are fundamentally relational beings. Healing and resilience are best forged through relational connections and social support (Shapiro, 2008). By sharing grief and ways to honor the deceased with kin and community, we regain our spirit to reengage fully with life and other relationships going forward.

NORMALIZING AND CONTEXTUALIZING COMPLICATED GRIEF PROCESSES

Extensive research finds that most bereaved persons experience transient and moderate distress over the early weeks and months after a death. Over time, the vast majority gradually adapt, returning to baseline levels of functioning, and many forge positive growth through the painful experience.

A small percentage of bereaved individuals (10–20%) suffer complicated grief, with a range of mental, physical, functional, and/or interpersonal impairments (Stroebe, Schut, & van den Bout, 2013). Research has focused mainly on individuals who suffer profound and persistent psychological distress in the loss of a significant dyadic bond. Studies find a heightened risk for poor physical health, shortened life expectancy, and suicide. Grief symptoms, such as yearning for the lost person and rumination about the death, often continue to dominate life, with the future seeming empty and bleak, and the person feeling lost and alone.

Based on studies of complicated grief in older widows and others who lost a significant attachment, Prigerson and colleagues proposed a new diagnostic category, prolonged grief disorder (PGD), which includes a range of symptomatic criteria (Prigerson, Kakarala, Gang, & Maciejewski, 2021). In 2013, the American Psychiatric Association adopted PGD as a new psychiatric condition in the fifth edition of the *Diagnostic and Statistical Manual of Mental Disorders* (DSM-5). PGD was also added to the *International Classification of Diseases* (ICD-11; World Health Organization, 2019; see Killikelly & Maercker, 2018). Both included grieving persons whose symptoms persisted longer than 6 months after a death. This provoked a backlash in a broader critique that mental health professionals were overdiagnosing and overmedicating patients (Kleinman, 2012), reviving a longstanding concern that grief not be treated as a disease (Engel, 1961).

In response, in 2022, the American Psychiatric Association revised its diagnostic criteria for PGD in DSM-5-TR. It now requires at least three of eight distressing mental and emotional symptoms for at least 12 months after the loss of a close attachment, with impairment in important areas of functioning (and distinct from major depressive disorder, posttraumatic stress disorder (PTSD), substance use, or other medical condition; Prigerson, Shear, & Reynolds, 2022). Prolonged grief disorder therapy (PGDT), a 16-week program of individual psychotherapy designed by M. K. Shear, focuses on symptoms concerning the lost bond, drawing on exposure techniques for victims of trauma for symptom reduction (Prigerson et al., 2022; Shear, 2015).

The diagnosis of PGD was intended to increase access to treatment for bereaved adults suffering a year after a loss (or at 6 months for youth) and unable to return to normal activities. However, the psychiatric classification of prolonged grief as a mental disorder poses several concerns for clinicians and for those needing help with bereavement. In the United States, the reimbursement system for psychotherapy is tied to managed care and the insurance industry, requiring a DSM diagnosis for coverage. With the DSM designation, clinicians can now bill insurance for treating people diagnosed with the condition. However, many who are in distress are reluctant to come for therapy with the stigma and shame of a psychiatric disorder. Having a diagnosis of mental disturbance on their permanent health records is also a serious concern. Yet, without the diagnosis, they may be denied coverage for loss-related issues. Clinicians sometimes use nonpathologizing diagnostic categories, such as reactive/adjustment disorder with anxiety or depression, but reimbursement may be denied if longer term therapy is needed.

A further concern is that the psychiatric diagnosis will lead to overmedicating the bereaved without attending to their loss experience and adaptational challenges. While short-term psychotropic drugs may be helpful in regaining daily functioning or reducing risks of self-harm, it's vital for clinicians to assess and address complex relational and contextual influences that may contribute to suffering and constrain adaptation. For instance, withdrawal into isolation, rumination, and despair after painful losses and the high risk of suicide are strongly influenced by social stigma and a lack of family and social support as well as by financial duress.

It's also problematic to define a certain length of time as a prolonged grief disorder. Setting a time limit implies that normal grief should be subsiding by this point and that further distress is abnormal. In a society that minimizes bereavement processes, it further stigmatizes grieving people who are encouraged to "get over it" as quickly as possible. Although the DSM adds that the duration and severity of the bereavement reaction should clearly exceed an individual's social, cultural, or religious norms, the criteria are based on American research and norms. Across and within cultures, there is tremendous diversity in what are considered normal mourning processes, such as length of time and emotional and behavioral expression. Gender and generational norms differ, and responses vary with the unique situations of a death, the relationship and role functioning lost, and the ramifications for survivors. The sudden death of a child, the loss of the family breadwinner, the destruction of homes and communities, or violent deaths in a car crash, homicide, or suicide are likely to pose more lengthy and complicated bereavement processes—which are normal (i.e., expectable, common, and understandable in context) in unexpected, extreme, or abnormal situations.

In sum, loss situations and grief and adaptation processes are varied and complex. A diagnosis of mental disorder and an arbitrary time frame for normal versus disordered grief don't account for the many influences that may contribute to distress and overwhelm functioning. Professionals need to be wary of any expectation that intense suffering should subside within a specific time. Moreover, clinicians need to be particularly alert to later bereavement complications that only arise long after a significant loss, as we found in our research and clinical experience (see, e.g., Walsh & McGoldrick, 2004). With the emotional upheaval of an unbearable loss or the press of immediate practical demands, initial grief may be submerged, only to surface in intense distress at an anniversary of the loss, another milestone, or in other relationships or life pursuits. Some persons come to therapy years later, presenting other mental or physical health concerns or relational or career problems that are related to a painful past loss, often not initially connecting their current difficulties to the earlier experience (see Chapter 10).

As Attig (2011) has cautioned, grieving is not about coming down with grief symptoms to be treated, and no one can grieve for us. More than painful reactions, the grieving response involves an active process in coping and relearning how to be and act in a world where loss transforms our lives. Loss forces us to relearn daily patterns and relationships with ourselves; with others, including the deceased; and with our faith; and to reexamine the meanings of our lives. Experiences with loss and grief are varied, complex, and richly textured. These life stories need to be understood for helping professionals to support clients' healing and resilience, soon after a loss or later in their life passage.

Understanding Traumatic Loss

The terms *trauma* and *traumatic* have become so widespread that they tend to be overgeneralized, often pathologizing normal or varied responses to sudden, extreme, or violent loss situations. Trauma literally means "wound, injury, or shock." A traumatic loss can refer to (1) an extreme and shocking death event, (2) an overwhelming experience, and/or (3) a debilitating personal reaction. Traumatic loss experiences can wound the mind, body, spirit, relationships with others, and future life pursuits. Trauma-informed individual approaches, combining cognitive-behavioral and exposure techniques, can be helpful in many cases (Perlman, Wortman, Feuer, Farber, & Rando, 2014).

Some loss events are so highly stressful that most people would find them traumatic, such as a violent death, murder, suicide, war, or widespread disaster. Yet there are considerable individual, relational, sociocultural, and contextual differences in impact. Too often, survivors are presumed to have PTSD, with faulty assumptions that most persons—adults or children—affected by the experience are likely to suffer profound and long-lasting damage.

Traumatic stress research has documented the human potential for recovery and resilience in a range of traumatic loss situations and social contexts. Studies of neurobiological and psychological processes show that acute stress symptoms are common in the immediate aftermath. Although some individuals are more vulnerable, no one is immune to suffering in extreme situations. Yet there is wide individual variation at the same level of risk: while up to a third experience long-term dysfunction, most distressed persons experience gradual recovery over time, and many forge remarkable resilience. Intense grief, suffering, and struggle to move forward often yield new strengths, transformation, and growth (Tedeschi, Shakespeare-Finch, Kanako, & Calhoun, 2018; see Chapter 2).

Healing and Treatment in Clinical Practice

Healing and treatment are distinct approaches in clinical practice. Western science, medicine, and psychotherapy have tended toward an unbalanced focus on pathology, with treatments designed and administered by experts and focused on symptom reduction. In addressing life-threatening conditions, metaphors of war and combat are prominent: winning or losing the battle, with aggressive treatments seen as weapons to destroy disease and conquer death.

Helping professionals foster healing through a collaborative therapeutic relationship that strengthens resources within the person, the family, and the community. Integrated biopsychosocial healthcare (McDaniel, Doherty, & Hepworth, 2013) focuses on the whole person and their loved ones and attends to influences in the family and larger systems to address suffering and foster well-being. Understanding systemic processes with an unbearable loss can enable clinicians to enhance functioning for healing and resilience.

Although psychotherapists are considered specialists in the healing art, some are uncomfortable with the notion of healing, in connotations of the therapist as healer, with the power to cure or alleviate pain, much like faith healers. Yet, in predominant treatment approaches over the past 50 years, therapists nonetheless assumed a position of authority over patients by virtue of their special knowledge, expertise, and professional status. Most therapy models have focused on therapist techniques to alter individual or family dysfunction. Strength-based systems approaches emphasize a therapeutic partnership that fosters clients' inherent potential for healing and resilience.

This collaborative approach is at the core of systemic practice in working with the dying and the bereaved. Distinct from curing or problem resolution, healing is seen as a natural systemic process in response to injury or trauma. One who is terminally ill may not recover physically, but they can heal mentally, emotionally, and spiritually in facing the end of life. Sometimes people heal physically but don't heal emotionally, mentally, or spiritually. The bereaved may return to basic functioning but don't regain the spirit to thrive or to fully love again; wounded relationships may remain unhealed. Therapists can foster psychosocial-spiritual healing even when a death cannot be reversed. The literal meaning of healing is becoming whole—and adapting and compensating for losses.

WORKING WITH INDIVIDUALS, COUPLES, AND FAMILIES: A RESILIENCE-ORIENTED SYSTEMIC PERSPECTIVE

This volume broadens our perspective on the experience of loss to understand individual symptoms in context and to consider the profound impact of loss in relational networks. It presents a resilience-oriented systemic approach to address complex situations of loss. As loved ones face end-of-life challenges and bereavement processes, we will see how their grief and adaptation can be complicated by many interacting influences: by the lack of preparation and sudden, unanticipated, or untimely occurrence of a loss; by the extreme or traumatic circumstances of a death; by complex family dynamics and past traumatic losses; and by unresponsive social contexts.

Adaptation to loss can be complicated by many factors. Grieving processes are especially challenging with ambiguous losses, as in the uncertain fate of a loved one or in the heartbreaking losses with dementia. Moreover, grief is hampered when it is unacknowledged, minimized, or stigmatized by others (see Chapters 7 and 8). Losses can be unbearable when violent or traumatic circumstances surround a death (see Chapter 9). Powerful emotional reactions, transmitted through emotional connections in relational systems, may find expression in other bonds (see Chapter 10). Unattended or suppressed grief may be distorted and displaced, becoming problematic in other relationships and life endeavors; it may be reactivated years later and across generations when the pain from past loss is aroused. In collective trauma events, loss and suffering are widespread, as in major disasters and pandemics; war and displacement; recurrent community violence; and mass shootings (see Chapter 11).

A resilience-oriented systemic assessment considers the sudden, violent, or traumatic nature and circumstances of a death; the emotional, practical, and social resources of the bereaved; and the multiple stressors and future challenges posed by the loss for individual, relational, and family functioning and well-being. In clinical work from a resilience perspective, we normalize grief as a universal experience in response to loss to reassure clients that distress is common; to respect cultural differences; and to expect varied reactions of family members, adults, and children. We strive to understand the complexities of their loss situation and the varying impact on their lives ahead. We attend to intense, persistent, or later symptoms, and we validate the distress without pathologizing it. The bereaved don't "get over" complicated and traumatic experiences of loss, but therapists can help them gradually come to terms with and weave them into the fabric of their lives going forward.

In the chapters that follow, we'll see how the impact of complex and traumatic loss experiences ripples throughout relational systems, touching all individuals and their bonds. Practice principles and case examples are offered to address pertinent issues, support grief processes, and strengthen capacities for resilience. The potential for healing and resilience depends greatly on the family response. Therefore, it's important for all mental health professionals, whether working with individuals, couples, or families, to understand and address the challenges and repercussions of complicated loss in relational networks. The family resilience framework described next, in Chapter 2, offers a useful guide to strengthen key relational processes that support healing and positive adaptation.

Working with Complex and Traumatic Loss

A Resilience-Oriented Systemic Approach

> Grief is in two parts. The first is loss.
> The second is the remaking of life.
> —ANNE ROIPHE, *Epilogue: A Memoir*

In helping clients facing the challenges of death and loss, a resilience-oriented systemic approach attends both to suffering and to pathways in grieving and positive adaptation. Therapy fosters healing and resilience by understanding the impact of loss in relational systems and social contexts, and mobilizing individual and relational processes and resources to support grieving and the ability to thrive beyond loss.

THE CONCEPT OF RESILIENCE: DYNAMIC SYSTEMIC PROCESSES

Resilience—the capacity to withstand and rebound from adversity—has become an important concept in mental health theory and research over recent decades. Most attention has focused on individual strengths in overcoming adverse life experiences. Many studies have addressed resilience in situations of complicated and traumatic loss (see, e.g., Bonanno, 2004; Walsh, 2007), as in the death of a child or in the wider impact of catastrophic events. More than weathering or surviving a tragic loss, resilience involves the process of coping and positive adaptation, regaining the ability to thrive, with the potential for personal and relational transformation and positive growth forged through the adverse experience. Similarly, studies of posttraumatic growth (PTG), an overlapping concept, have found that many persons who suffered and struggled experienced positive personal transformation beyond recovery (Tedeschi et al., 2018). They developed increased appreciation of life, deeper relational bonds, more meaningful priorities, enhanced sense of personal strength, realization of new possibilities and pathways in life, and new or renewed spiritual development.

Advances in research have expanded our understanding of human resilience to recognize that it involves multilevel systemic processes in the dynamic interplay of individual, family, community, institutional, sociocultural, and environmental influences in our social ecology (Masten, 2019; Ungar, 2020). The family as an adaptive system and the primary context for human development plays a central role in risk and resilience in situations of adversity. In this volume, we focus on understanding couple and family challenges and resilience with death, dying, and loss because of their crucial importance for both individual and relational healing and growth. This chapter describes a family systems perspective and identifies key interactional processes in relational systems that clinicians can facilitate for individual, couple, and family resilience in the experience of loss.

A FAMILY SYSTEMS ORIENTATION

A relational view of human resilience recognizes the significance of supportive relationships in positive adaptation for individuals facing death and loss. A family systems orientation expands our understanding to the ongoing mutuality of influences in the relational network. More than the problems or support of individual family members, a systemic perspective attends to risk and resilience in the family as a functional unit, affecting all members and their bonds.

Beyond coping and adaptation, mourning processes can yield both personal and relational transformation and positive growth. *New York Times* columnist Charles Blow wrote of the powerful impact of the death of his older brother at age 58 from complications of chronic medical conditions (Blow, 2020). He was astonished by the outpouring of support in his childhood hometown:

> The community will not allow you to grieve in solitude. They are there, encircling you, holding you, lifting you. Everyone brings something. Many sit and talk for a bit, some sharing a laugh, some shedding a tear. Your sorrow is shared sorrow; the weight on your shoulders is shared by many.

Over the following year Blow experienced a profound personal transformation (Blow, 2022):

> My brother's death blew a hole in me and made me reconsider everything.
> "What kind of life did I want to live? What kind of man—kind of person—
> did I want to be?" Within a month, I changed everything. I stopped drink-
> ing. I learned to sit with myself, alone, and experience my emotions, and to
> deal with tough days, and even the exhilarating ones, head on. I was, and
> am, still dating someone truly special who has taught me what being at peace
> with yourself looks like.
>   And I have come to see things clearly again—things that seem so sim-
> ple to me now, but that somehow I couldn't see then: that life is a series of
> peaks and valleys, and it is a fool's errand to try to flatten them out. That
> beauty is in the connections we make, to self, to family, to friends, to the
> earth. That we don't judge the quality of a life by the volume at which we
> live it. That I deserve to be kind to myself.

In my own research and practice, I have been inspired by the strengths
and potential forged by so many bereaved loved ones after tragic loss.
Through their experience of deep suffering and support, they became
more resilient, rebuilding their lives, strengthening bonds, and regaining
the ability to thrive. For instance, the death of a child heightens risk for
marital distancing and divorce; yet, with mutual support through the tragedy, couples and families often emerge from painful losses stronger and
more resourceful in meeting challenges (Greeff & Human, 2004; Greeff,
Vansteenwegen, & Herbiest, 2011; Stinnett & DeFrain, 1985). Family
members often develop new insights and abilities, reappraise life priorities, and become committed to new purpose in memory of the deceased.
A death or threatened loss can heighten appreciation of loved ones and
spur efforts to repair grievances. Past experiences, stories, and role models
of courage, tenacity, and ingenuity in dealing with other adversities can
inspire efforts in facing new challenges.

Family resilience refers to relational capacities as a functional system to
withstand and rebound from adverse life events and loss experiences. A
basic systems premise is that a significant loss impacts the whole family;
in turn, how the family deals with the loss facilitates the adaptation of all
members, their relationships, and the family unit. In practice, a resilience-
oriented approach (1) attends with compassion to the challenges, suffering, and struggles of clients; and (2) identifies and builds on relational
processes and social resources that support grief processes, coping, and
positive adaptation. With a multisystemic lens, it draws on extended kin
and social support and on community, larger systems, sociocultural, and
spiritual resources (see Figure 2.1).

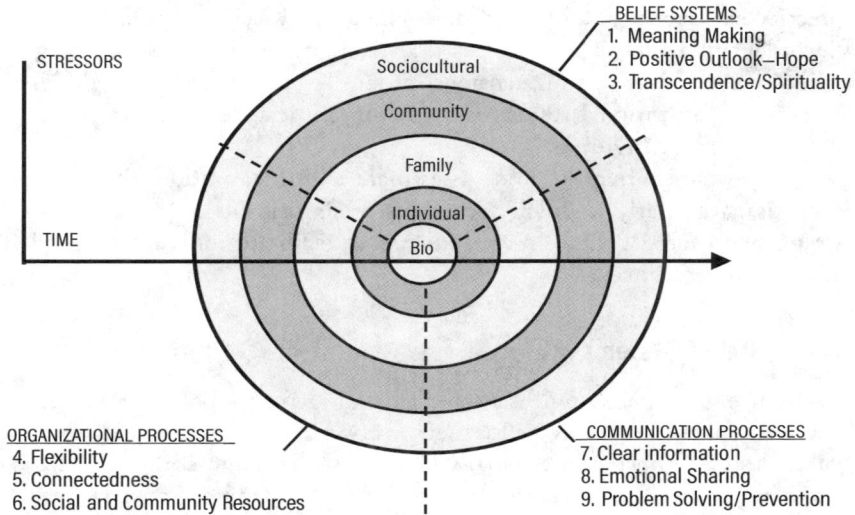

Belief Systems
1. Meaning Making
2. Positive Outlook–Hope
3. Transcendence/Spirituality

Organizational Processes
4. Flexibility
5. Connectedness
6. Social and Community Resources

Communication Processes
7. Clear information
8. Emotional Sharing
9. Problem Solving/Prevention

FIGURE 2.1. Multilevel systemic processes in resilience. From Walsh (2016b). Copyright © 2016 The Guilford Press. Reprinted by permission.

In all situations of death and loss, grief and adaptation may be complicated by unhelpful relational processes in couple and family systems. Beyond family borders, social, educational, workplace, legal, and community systems impact bereavement processes. A lack of emotional and practical support or multistress obstacles in rebuilding lives, such as financial security after the death of a breadwinner or a pileup of medical bills, can complicate recovery from a devastating loss. In sum, a systemic approach to practice strives to understand and situate each person's experience of loss and grief processes in their family and social context. Our aim is to normalize and contextualize extreme distress as understandable in complex and traumatic situations of death and loss.

APPLYING A FAMILY RESILIENCE FRAMEWORK

A family resilience framework integrates ecosystemic and developmental dimensions of experience. Powerful social influences are not simply external forces or factors that impact families. Understood in dynamic terms, families counter risks and mobilize resources as members navigate challenges in their social environment.

The Walsh Family Resilience Framework, grounded in extensive practice experience and research on resilience and well-functioning families, identified nine key processes that facilitate family resilience, organized in three domains (dimensions) of family functioning: shared belief systems, organizational resources, and communication processes (Walsh, 2003, 2016c; see Figure 2.2).

As a practice map to guide assessment and intervention, this framework is particularly useful in situations of significant loss to target and strengthen shared beliefs and practices that facilitate individual, couple, and family resilience.

Family Belief Systems

Each family's belief system is rooted in multigenerational, sociocultural, and spiritual influences, as well as their position in their social world. Shared values and assumptions are socially constructed through core convictions and ongoing transactions that powerfully shape members' approaches to death and their pathways in adaptation to loss. In turn, core beliefs may be disrupted or modified by significant loss experiences. Because family beliefs come to the fore in complex loss situations, heightened attention is given to key resilience-promoting beliefs and practices in (1) meaning making, (2) a positive outlook, and (3) transcendence and spirituality.

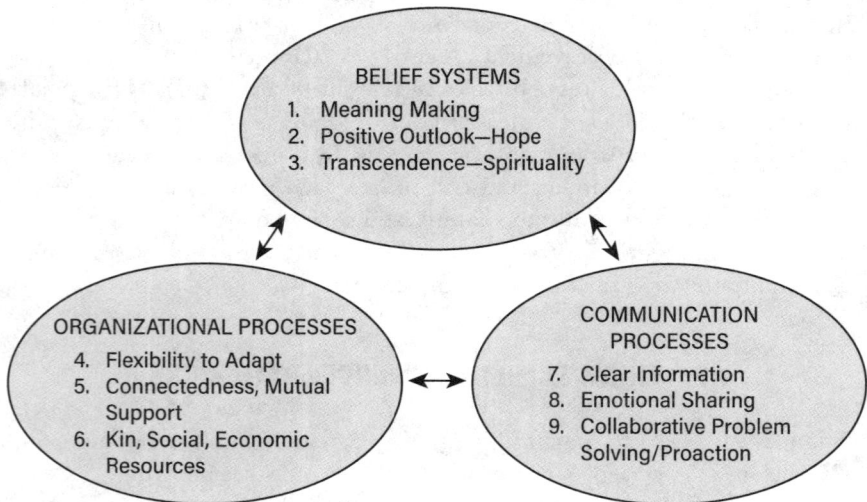

FIGURE 2.2. Key processes in family resilience. From Walsh (2016b). Copyright © 2016 The Guilford Press. Reprinted by permission.

Meaning Making

Meaning making occurs through the narratives we construct to make sense of our world and our position in it. Meaning-making processes are significant in the experience of loss, particularly with the death of a significant person and when it occurs tragically or prematurely (Neimeyer, Klass, & Dennis, 2014). It can shake the foundations of our assumptive and relational world and lead to anguished attempts to find meaning in the loss and in our lives in its aftermath. This struggle can yield positive growth (Neimeyer, Bottomley, & Bellet, 2018).

A systems perspective views meaning-making processes as socially constructed: nurtured, sustained, and altered through dynamic transactional processes in significant relational systems. Family and cultural history and values, as well as community and larger societal influences, play a role. Accounts may initially seem chaotic and conflict with the perspectives of others in their relational system. Stories of loss often evolve over time as people grapple with its meaning and impact or gain new information or insights.

In families, meaning-making processes involve shared attempts to make sense of a death and loss, put it in perspective to make it more bearable, and gradually integrate it into life passage (Hooghe & Neimeyer, 2013; Nadeau, 1997, 2008). Meaning-making processes are ongoing—not some final wrap-up at the "end" of a mourning process that "makes sense" of a loss. They begin in initial attempts to explain what has happened and how it occurred. Family members commonly grapple with painful questions such as: "Why us?" "Why my child [parent or spouse]?" "Why not me?" They ask, "How can we go on?" Understandings shift or deepen with new information and perspectives; other meanings emerge as they grapple with future ramifications. And families construct stories of their loss to tell others and gain narrative coherence of their experience.

Family resilience is strengthened through shared efforts to gain a *sense of coherence*: recasting the loss situation (what happened to them) as shared challenges that are comprehensible, manageable, and meaningful to tackle (Antonovsky & Sourani, 1988). Families need to hold and integrate multiple meanings of a loss, with different implications for various members, bonds, and role functioning. For instance, in one single-parent family, with the death of the mother's brother, her son lost his special bond with his uncle, who was like his "second dad" after his father left.

Causal attributions concerning blame, shame, and guilt are especially strong when questions of personal responsibility, fault, or negligence arise. Family members may become preoccupied with thoughts that they or others could have or should have done something to prevent a death. It is important to help them share such concerns and come to terms with any accountability as well as the limits of control in their situation. A traumatic loss situation can shatter core assumptions concerning normalcy, predictability, and security (Janoff-Bulman, 1992; see Chapters 9–12). Coming to terms with a "senseless" death, as in a random event or an incomprehensible suicide, can be especially painful, with prolonged rumination common and the need to accept ambiguity in some situations. Still, a meaningful response—making meaning through purposeful action from a senseless death—can foster healing.

With the disruptions wrought by death, efforts in meaning reconstruction promote healing (Neimeyer & Sands, 2011). Coming to terms with loss involves finding ways to weave the experience into the fabric of both individual and relational life passages. Clinicians can support family efforts to comprehend the loss—including its lingering questions and its ongoing and future implications—and gradually to place it in some meaningful perspective that fits coherently with their life experience and aspirations. Therapists should be cautious not to ascribe meaning to clients' unique experience; the therapeutic role is not to *provide* meaning but to facilitate their meaning-making process (Frankl, 1946/2006).

A Positive Outlook

Abundant research attests to the importance of a positive outlook for resilience. Yet this should not be seen as relentless optimism and good cheer. Resilience is most often forged through suffering and struggle. In recovering from a significant loss, everyone at times falters and experiences setbacks. As one bereaved mother said, "You fall down five times but get up six times."

Sustaining hope is most essential in times of deepest despair. Hope might be thought of as oxygen for the spirit, fueling energies and efforts to cope and adapt. Weingarten (2010) stresses the importance of practicing reasonable hope, reorienting what is hoped for, as when facing a grim prognosis with a life-threatening condition (see Chapter 4).

Normalizing and contextualizing distress as common and understandable in devastating loss situations can depathologize family members' varied reactions and reduce blame, shame, and guilt. This is especially important with regard to the psychiatric diagnosis of intense and persistent grief as PGD (see Chapter 1). Affirming relational strengths amid difficulties counters a sense of helplessness, failure, and despair as it reinforces shared pride, confidence, and a "can do" spirit. Family members' mutual encouragement bolsters members' efforts to take initiative and persevere in efforts to cope and overcome challenges.

Active agency in *mastering the possible* is crucial for resilience: focusing on what can be done, accepting what can't be changed or is beyond control, and tolerating uncertainty. Those who are contending with a terminal illness may despair that, despite best efforts, optimism, prayers, or medical care, they can't avert death. Clinicians can help them to reorient hope: to shift focus from an outcome beyond their control to make the most of precious time, alleviate suffering, and heal relational grievances (see Chapter 4). In the wake of loss, families cannot bring a loved one back to life or change the circumstances of a death—nor can clinicians. When I met with one couple who had recently lost their child to cancer, the father cried out, "I don't know why we're seeing you—you can't bring back our son!" Yet we can support the bereaved in their grief and encourage their efforts to find renewed meaning and purpose. When death shatters future hopes and dreams, therapists can help family members to reorient their lives and reenvision possibilities.

Transcendent Values and Spirituality

Transcendent values and practices help families face death and loss, connecting personal tragedy and suffering with our common humanity. They expand the perspective of immediate suffering as part of a larger, meaningful whole in life passage and in the human condition.

Clinicians are encouraged to attend to the spiritual dimension of experience with death, dying, and loss as spiritual matters commonly come to the fore during these times (see Chapter 3). As Wright and Bell (2021) have observed, suffering invites us into the spiritual domain. It's important to explore any spiritual concerns that contribute to distress and to identify spiritual resources, fitting clients' orientation, that might support their healing and resilience.

Death ends a life, but relationships are sustained through ongoing spiritual and symbolic connections, transmitted through memories, stories, and deeds. Many find solace in their belief that a tragic death may be beyond human comprehension but part of God's larger plan or a test of faith. Those who believe in a spiritual afterlife may find comfort in viewing death as a passage to another realm. Those who are not religious may find benefit in discussing existential concerns about the meaning of their lives.

Religious concerns can be a major source of distress (see Chapter 3). In one case, a husband secretly believed that the couple's infertility was God's punishment for his past infidelity. Some are in anguish when a death seems unjust, shattering their faith in God, or when prayers for a miracle were not answered. Consultation/collaboration with pastoral professionals may be helpful in such situations.

Transcendent beliefs and practices that fit with clients' religious or secular values can foster resilience at times of death and loss (see Chapter 3). Spiritual nourishment may be found within and outside organized religion: through deep faith and/or congregational support; contemplative practices; and connectedness with nature. The expressive arts, as in writing, music, drama, or art, can foster healing resilience following unbearable loss (Saul, 2013; Thompson & Neimeyer, 2014). Many families surmount heartbreaking loss by helping others in community service or social actions to alleviate or prevent suffering or address harmful conditions.

Beyond coping and adaptation, the suffering and struggle with loss can yield personal and relational transformation and growth in couples and families, similar to the findings of posttraumatic growth for individuals (Tedeschi et al., 2018). Members develop new insights and abilities, reappraising and redirecting life priorities. A death or threatened loss can heighten appreciation of surviving loved ones and spur efforts to repair grievances. Family histories, stories, and role models of courage, tenacity, and ingenuity in dealing with painful losses or other adversity offer inspiration to surmount overwhelming tragedy.

Organizational Resources

The shock and pain of loss disrupts family functioning and can shatter cohesion, leaving members to fend for themselves, isolated in their grief, as occurred in Zoe's family after the mother's death (see Chapter 1). Reorganizing adaptive patterns of interaction can facilitate healing and resilience for all members and the family unit. Key processes involve (1) flexibility; (2) connectedness; and (3) extended kinship, social, and economic resources.

Flexibility to Adapt and Reorganize

Family organization requires flexibility to adapt to the changes wrought by loss and to restabilize in its aftermath. In navigating disruptive changes, families need to reorganize patterns of interaction, with strong leadership to provide continuity, security, and dependability for children and other vulnerable family members. Clear leadership roles, rules, and routines are important. It is helpful to inquire about what changed in family life with a death. We might ask about a typical day and/or a typical week before and since the loss. Often, in the chaotic aftermath, there is no typical day or week, so families may need help in reestablishing basic functioning in everyday life in the short term, with later renegotiation for long-term adaptation.

We explore family relationship and role realignments with the loss. Families may need help in rebuilding or transferring the authoritative leadership necessary to manage the disruptive aftermath and carry on. The impact is greater when the loss is that of important role functioning, as with the death of a primary breadwinner, parent, or caregiver. A son or daughter may be called upon to set aside their own priorities to assume caregiving functions or to earn needed family income. Clinicians can facilitate discussions to brainstorm functional arrangements to carry on, while considering the needs and priorities of all members.

Family functioning can become disorganized following a significant loss, especially with a pileup of stressors. Families risk a cascade of destabilizing changes, as when a residential relocation generates other losses and adjustments, especially for children. A family may benefit from coaching to pace and buffer disruptions, supporting children and vulnerable family members. At the other extreme, a family can become frozen in time if surviving members aren't able to reallocate role functions and reconfigure relational bonds. An overly rigid family may need help in modifying set patterns and in making necessary accommodations to loss (see Chapter 5).

Connectedness

Building connectedness through teamwork and mutual support is essential for resilience. All relationships experience occasional conflict, mixed feelings, or shifting alliances. The shock and pain of loss can shatter family cohesion, leaving members to fend for themselves, isolated in their grief. The mourning process tends to be more complicated if there has been intense or persistent conflict, relational abuse, strong ambivalence, or estrangement (see Chapter 10). When differences are viewed as disloyal and threatening, members may submerge or distort feelings or turn against one another. The common idealization of the deceased can provoke outrage and alienation by a child who suffered abuse by the parent who died. Some members distance, with emotional and physical cutoffs. One son, age 18, unable to tolerate his family's intense grief after the father's death, abruptly left home and moved across the country, saying he took "the geographic cure." When death is anticipated, it is important to encourage family members to (re)connect and take steps to repair strained relationships before the opportunity is lost (see Chapter 4).

Extended Family, Social, and Economic Resources

It is crucial to mobilize extended family, social, and community networks for both practical and emotional support. Family recovery is imperiled

when finances are drained by costly, protracted medical care or the loss
of a vital breadwinner. It is important to help families discuss financial
concerns, which may be shame-laden and hidden, especially for widowed elders. Structural supports provided by larger systems, such as paid
bereavement leave and quality, affordable child and elder care, are also
crucial for families to make time and space for mourning processes. Too
many families lack such benefits, which complicates their grieving and
adaptation.

Communication Processes

When a family confronts a painful loss, open communication facilitates
the processes of meaning making, reorganization, emotional support, and
problem solving going forward.

Clear Information

Family grief processes and resilience are supported by clear, consistent
information about the loss situation and future expectations. Clinicians
can facilitate efforts to clarify the facts and circumstances of a death and
consider how and with whom to share them. In situations where the cause
of death is unclear, it is particularly important to support family efforts to
gain information from healthcare providers or the appropriate authorities. Often, only a spouse, a primary caregiver, or a family representative
is given information; they may be in shock and distraught, and unsure
how and with whom to share details. Family members often have different understandings, based on fragmentary or conflicting information and
depending on their ages and level of cognitive understanding.

Open Emotional Sharing

Open emotional sharing with empathic response facilitates grief processes
and strengthens bonds. It is important to foster a relational climate of
mutual trust, empathic response, and tolerance for a wide range and fluctuation of responses over time. Emotional reactions will vary with one's
relationship with the deceased and implications of the loss; with individual coping styles; with a child's developmental phase; with different
pacing in recovery; and with role functioning and demands of other life
challenges. At different moments, strong emotions may surface, including complicated and mixed feelings of anger, disappointment, helplessness, relief, guilt, and abandonment. In couples, emotional attunement is

important, especially when partners differ in how they are expressing their grief (Hooghe, Rosenblatt, & Rober, 2017).

It is important to rekindle warm interactions in sharing positive feelings, mutual appreciation, and enjoyable times together, which can get lost in the midst of grief. Clinicians need to rebalance a commonly skewed therapeutic overfocus on the painful emotions and symptom reduction that bring people to therapy. Sharing moments of joy, gratitude, fun, and humor in therapy sessions and in family life offers respite from suffering and struggle, revitalizing energies and bonds.

Collaborative Problem Solving and Planning Steps Ahead

Clinicians can be helpful in facilitating family discussion, brainstorming, and collaboration on coping strategies and decision making. When overwhelmed by loss-related challenges, it's important to support incremental steps and to celebrate small successes, expecting inevitable mistakes and setbacks, and viewing them as learning opportunities. In gaining new confidence and competencies through their efforts, families become more resourceful. Therapists also need to support efforts to shift from a crisis-reactive mode to future-oriented planning: anticipating and preparing to meet adaptive challenges ahead.

Dynamic Interplay of Relational Processes

In helping individuals, couples, and families facing death and loss, a number of studies show the benefit in applying a family resilience framework and in targeting these key transactional processes to strengthen individual and relational resilience. Barboza and colleagues (Barboza & Seedall, 2021; Barboza, Seedall, & Neimeyer, 2022) found that these key processes in families were associated with reduced severity in grief-related symptoms of individual members by actively supporting their adaptive meaning-making processes.

These transactional processes involve beliefs and skills that therapists can help couples and families to mobilize and strengthen. The nine key processes are mutually interactive and synergistic, building on each other. Effective communication facilitates meaning making and family organizational flexibility. In turn, meaning making, flexibility, and collaboration facilitate problem-solving steps going forward. Key processes may be expressed in various ways, related to cultural norms and family preferences. Some may be more (or less) relevant in different situations of loss and with evolving challenges over time. As bereaved families cope and adapt, they forge varying pathways in resilience depending on their values and aims.

PRINCIPLES OF RESILIENCE-ORIENTED SYSTEMIC PRACTICE

A family resilience orientation is finding broad application in strength-based, collaborative, systemic practice, policy, and research (Walsh, 2016a, 2016c). Risk and resilience in adaptation to loss are viewed in light of multiple, mutual influences involving biological, psychological, family, social, community, larger systems, and cultural/spiritual variables.

A resilience-oriented systemic approach attends to grief processes, risks for maladaptation, and relational processes that foster positive adaptation, strengthening the family and its members for their future life passage. It emphasizes collaborative processes and seeks to identify and build on strengths and resources. This approach is broadly inclusive of sociocultural, developmental, and multigenerational influences in vulnerability, risk, and resilience. Intervention efforts aim to enhance family coping, mastery, and growth in dealing with loss-related life challenges. Practice principles are outlined in Table 2.1.

A family resilience orientation can be usefully applied in all strength-based, systemic practices whether working with individuals, couples, or families. This approach to loss requires therapists to show the same flexibility that families themselves need to respond to various members' priorities and concerns that come to the fore. Decisions to meet with children or adult family members or to hold couples or whole family sessions at various points are guided by a systemic view of bereavement processes, fitting emerging priorities. This approach attends with compassion when

---

TABLE 2.1. Resilience-Oriented Systemic Perspective with Loss-Related Challenges

- Relational view of human resilience
- Grounded in developmental systemic perspective
- Biopsychosocial–cultural–spiritual influences
- Shift from deficit view of loss-related distress to challenge by complicated loss experience
  - ♦ with focus on healing and positive adaptation
- Significant loss impacts the family system; family response influences
  - ♦ the adaptation of all members, relationships, and family unit
- Contextual view of crisis, symptoms of distress, and adaptation
  - ♦ Family, social, and cultural–spiritual influences
  - ♦ Developmental/temporal influences
    - ◊ Timing of symptoms and loss events
    - ◊ Pileup of stressors, persistent adversity
    - ◊ Adaptational challenges over time
    - ◊ Individual and family developmental phases
    - ◊ Anniversary, multigenerational patterns

painful emotions are aroused, and it encourages active steps that facilitate mourning and adaptational processes over time. As I have seen time and again, our clients' remarkable resilience can emerge through our collaborative work.

A systemic assessment takes a broadly inclusive view of the family (see Chapter 1). We attend to the multiple influences in bereavement throughout the relational network, including important roles and relationships within and beyond households, biological and step-relations, and informal kinship bonds. The genogram and timeline (McGoldrick, Gerson, & Petry, 2020) can guide family inquiry and intervention planning by visualizing and tracking family dynamics, structural patterns, relational resources, major events, and past, recent, and threatened loss experiences. Therapists should evaluate the general level of family functioning, the current state of relationships, changes with a death, and challenges ahead. We identify potential resources in the extended family, social, and community network. It is important to explore (1) the impact of the death and loss on the family system, its members, and their relationships; and (2) the family approach to the loss situation. Interventions utilize principles and techniques that are common among strength-based family systems approaches, while they attend more centrally to the impact of significant losses and other stressors on family life and aim to increase family capacities for positive adaptation.

A family systemic assessment may lead to individual, couple, family, and/or group modalities. Family consultations, brief intervention, or more intensive family therapy may be indicated. Individual therapy may include conjoint sessions, inviting others most affected by the loss and those who may be constraining and/or might support healing and resilience. Therapy with an individual following spousal or child loss might include one or more parent–child sessions or meetings for the sibling group. Since therapy contact may be brief, while grief and restoration processes are likely to be lengthy, it might be helpful to hold brief "well-being checkups" at the time of stressful transitions, such as the first anniversary of a death, or with emerging challenges in long-term adaptation.

Resilience-oriented services like these foster family empowerment as they bring forth shared hope, develop new and renewed competencies, and strengthen family bonds. Interventions to strengthen family resilience also have preventive value, building capacities in meeting future challenges. Further, studies have found that in focusing on client resilience, helping professionals working with trauma experienced *vicarious resilience* in their work, countering burnout and yielding greater personal, relational, and spiritual well-being in their own lives (Hernandez, Engstrom, & Gangsei, 2010; see Chapter 12).

Caution is required to ensure that the concept of family resilience is not misapplied, leading one to judge or label families or their members as "not resilient" or "too dysfunctional" if they have prolonged difficulty in recovering from tragic loss situations. Family processes can strengthen coping and adaptive capacities, and yet they may not be sufficient to overcome devastating biological, social, or environmental conditions. Just as the resilience of an individual is not limited to the capacities that a person can muster alone, so too, the resilience of the family depends on supports by interconnected larger systems for grieving losses and rebuilding lives. To bolster the resilience of multistressed families and underresourced communities, a multilevel approach requires attention to barriers and supports for bereaved families and their members to thrive.

Throughout this volume, we'll apply the principles and guidelines of a resilience-oriented systemic approach in practice to help clients who are struggling with a range of challenges in complex and traumatic loss situations.

CHAPTER 3

Cultural and Spiritual Influences in Suffering, Healing, and Resilience

Death is only a horizon.
And a horizon is nothing save the limit of our sight.
—WILLIAM PENN

People over the ages have turned to cultural and spiritual resources to cope with the precariousness of life, the disruptions wrought by death, and the mystery of the beyond. While death and loss are universal human experiences, varied belief systems approach the end of life and mourning processes in their own ways. Each offers a worldview that helps people face the inescapable fact of death, including the rhythms of life and an abiding faith in some continuity beyond death.

MULTICULTURAL AND INTERGENERATIONAL PERSPECTIVES

Helping individuals and families face death and loss requires our understanding of their cultural beliefs and norms, as well as differences across generations and social contexts.

In *The Farewell*, a film based on a true story (Wang, 2019), Billi, a Chinese American young artist living in New York, learns that her beloved grandmother, Nai-Nai, the family matriarch, is dying. The extended family members are gathering in China to see her one last time. When informed by the doctor that Nai-Nai has terminal lung cancer and is expected to live only a few months, they agree to keep the diagnosis a secret from her. They schedule an impromptu fake wedding as an excuse for their gathering. They worry that Billi, raised with American values, will expose the lie to her grandmother.

Billi clashes with the family over their dishonesty. She believes that a terminally ill person should be told the truth to respect her right to know and to give her the chance to say her final good-byes and put her affairs in order. Her uncle tells her that their way, based in ancient Chinese cultural values, differs from the truth-telling, individualistic values of Western culture. From their perspective, the lie allows the family to bear the emotional burden of the prognosis, sparing Nai-Nai from distress and instead enabling her to share happiness with them in what short time remains. Billi agrees to keep the secret. She later learns that Nai-Nai also told a similar lie to her husband when he was terminally ill.

As the film's ending credits reveal, the woman Nai-Nai's character was based upon was still alive—6 years after her fatal diagnosis.

Cultural beliefs, family norms, and intergenerational relations are interconnected. Traditional values may be problematic for younger generations in diverse and rapidly changing societies. A recent study in mainland China (Li, Chan, & Marrable, 2023) found that complex intergenerational family dynamics hampered the adaptation of adolescents and emerging adults who had lost a parent. Family bereavement processes, strongly influenced by Confucian beliefs and cultural traditions, discouraged the sharing of information, acknowledgment, and emotional expression of grief (considered crucial tasks for adaptation in Western culture; see Chapter 4). Family members excluded them from medical information and family decisions during their parent's dying process. An implicit family rule constructed by the surviving parent and extended family discouraged grieving openly, with no grief-related conversation permitted. This isolated the bereaved young person and disenfranchised their grief interpersonally and socially. Their attempts were not successful in emotionally reinvesting in other relationships, especially with the surviving parent.

Complications were more likely when the loss coincided with other family-level maladaptive copings, such as the surviving parent's precipitous remarriage, which in turn disrupted family cohesion. Thus, the young person often ruminated over their loss experience and struggled over time, searching for understanding and support.

In working with loss and grief, it's essential to understand cultural mourning processes in developmental and social contexts, to explore each person's subjective perspective, and to avoid stereotypic assumptions. As we've already seen, there may be important differences in values, needs, and life experience within cultures and families.

ADDRESSING CONSTRAINTS OF GENDER-BASED SOCIALIZATION

As gender identity, roles, and relationships have become more varied in recent decades, traditional gender-based norms in bereavement widely persist. Women are more often expected to handle social, emotional, and caregiving demands, from expressing grief to caring for the terminally ill and surviving family members, including a spouse's extended family. Men, socialized to manage instrumental tasks, are most often expected to take charge of funeral and financial arrangements.

Cultural images of strong masculinity commonly constrain men from sharing "soft" emotions in grief; many are reluctant to look weak by revealing vulnerability or dependency. They are more likely to express anger than sorrow and to withdraw, seek refuge in their work, or turn to alcohol, drugs, or an affair. This response constrains both their seeking and giving of emotional support. With a tragic loss, women are more likely to seek professional help and to acknowledge distress. Since mothers are expected to protect their children, they more often feel they are at fault for a pregnancy loss or they are seen as responsible for a child's death. Partners' different responses to loss can strain couple relationships. Many men are uncomfortable with their loved one's expressions of grief, are unsure how to respond, and fear losing control of their own feelings (culturally framed as "breaking down" or "falling apart"). Professionals may need to work harder to engage men in therapy when the need for help is seen as a sign of weakness, inadequacy, or a mental disorder.

Sharlayne, age 43, was in individual therapy for several months, with inconsolable grief after her only child, 18-year-old Jimmy, had collapsed and died in her arms. Sharlayne and James, Sr., a Black working-class couple, had struggled to raise Jimmy well and were proud that he had just earned a scholarship to college. Although James, too, had lost his only child, and his namesake, he refused therapy for himself, balking at the clinic's symptom checklist and implications that there was something wrong with him. He said he was fine and didn't need any help. His stoic manner of maintaining control was a source of pride for him.

As a consultant, I asked the therapist if James might be willing to come to a few sessions with his wife to support her recovery. The therapist replied, "Well—he drives her to every session and waits for her in the car." James agreed, with the therapist's encouragement that he could be helpful by sitting by her side in sessions and by sharing his own views. Soon James gained trust in the therapist and unburdened his own deep pain, and both spouses found comfort in sharing their grief and in their mutual support.

It's important to normalize vulnerability and grief as inherent in our human condition, emphasizing that it takes strength and courage to show deep emotions and vulnerabilities. We can also encourage involvement by tapping into a deep desire to be a responsible and loving partner or a strong role model for children. Yet, men socialized as problem solvers may feel helpless when they can't "fix" or "solve" a tragic loss situation. A grieving spouse may perceive their partner's emotional unavailability as abandonment when they need comfort most, thereby experiencing a double loss.

Elena came for individual therapy, despondent for many months over the sudden death of her brother and unable to attend to housework and child care. Her husband, Carlos, in frustration that she wasn't "getting over it," distanced from her, increasing her sense of isolation and despair.

In a couple consultation session, Elena sat hunched over, crying softly into tissues. Carlos sat apart from her, on the sidelines of her grief and her therapy. Carlos, a construction worker, said he felt helpless when she cried and was at a loss about what to do—he couldn't "fix it." Asked what he meant, he said, "I can't bring back her brother!" At my suggestion, he asked Elena how he could be more supportive. She replied, "Just hold me." Carlos looked stunned. "That's all you need me to do?" "Yes, please, hold me tight." Carlos pulled his chair up close and wrapped his arms around her as she wept into his chest. The therapist likened his support to the sturdy beams that hold up a house being repaired after a devastating storm.

With the therapist's encouragement, Elena added, "My big brother was always there for me when we were kids. I feel so alone. I need to know you'll be here for me—that you won't leave me, too." Carlos assured her of his love and commitment. Over the following weeks, the idea of "doing support" was expanded to flexibly alter family role functioning to share more household and child care tasks and to have their children contribute to the teamwork. Surprising the parents, they didn't resist, instead feeling better to be included in restoring family life.

INTERTWINING OF CULTURAL AND SPIRITUAL INFLUENCES

Spiritual beliefs and practices are interwoven with sociocultural influences. In contrast to the individualism of the dominant American society, most cultural and spiritual orientations worldwide see meaningful human experience as embedded in family, the larger community, and wider circles of connection. In ancient Indigenous worldviews, life is a cycle of birth, death, and rebirth; the spirit never dies, and just as in physics, energy is never destroyed, only transformed. Ancestors, though no longer physically present, can still communicate with loved ones and descendants, acting as spiritual guardians.

Recent Latinx and other immigrants commonly value traditional cultural and spiritual resources when facing death and loss (Falicov, 2014, 2016). Some follow ancient beliefs and practices alongside Western medicine and their Christian faith, turning to the church for funerals, yet maintaining special relationships with spiritual guides, shamans, and rituals. Incense, candles, crystals, sacred objects, herbal remedies, and potions may be used to cure illness and ward off death. Many believe in an invisible world inhabited by good and evil spirits who can protect or harm, bring good luck or misfortune, and prevent or cause death. Sudden death or life-threatening illness may be seen as due to possession by harmful spirits. Many believe that they can communicate directly with the spirits of ancestors, who, if honored appropriately, will confer their blessings and protection. It's common in many cultures to experience spiritual visitations, divine healing, or miracles; transpersonal encounters with angels or demons; and direct contact and conversation with deceased loved ones.

In the annual Mexican tradition of the Día de los Muertos (Day of the Dead), altars (offrendas) are decorated with flowers, photos, and memorabilia to honor deceased loved ones at home, in public spaces, and at cemeteries. Offerings to the departed are set out in miniature replicas of their loved ones' favorite foods and beverages or in toys for a deceased child. In cemeteries, one can see elaborately constructed altars at gravesites surrounded by candles to light the way for the nighttime return of their loved ones' spirit. The next day, family members, young and old, gather for a graveside feast, welcoming back the souls of the departed. I was once invited to witness this deeply moving tradition with a Mexican research psychologist. She told me that at each celebration she experiences the presence of her deceased father, which gives her the strength to overcome difficulties in the year to come.

Clinicians should be mindful not to superimpose a Western cultural and scientific or a Judeo-Christian template on other belief systems and practices. It's important to ask clients about traditional ways, which may not be mentioned, as they have often been demeaned as primitive or contact with the deceased has been diagnosed as delusional (Falicov, 2014).

ADDRESSING THE SPIRITUAL DIMENSION

Spiritual beliefs commonly come to the fore when facing death and loss. Yet many clinicians are ill equipped by their training or are hesitant to ask about spiritual matters (see Chapter 12). Just as we would explore cultural influences, it's important to attend to the spiritual dimension of clients' experience with loss: (1) to understand the meaning and significance of their spiritual beliefs and practices, (2) to explore any spiritual sources of distress, and (3) to draw on potential spiritual resources for healing and resilience.

It's important to distinguish the overlapping concepts of religion and spirituality (R/S), which are often mistakenly polarized or conflated (Walsh, 2009d). Religion refers to an organized faith system, with shared doctrines, practices, and a community of followers. Religions provide moral values, beliefs about God or a Higher Power, and congregational affiliation for a spiritual home, pastoral guidance, and support. Sacred texts, teachings, rituals, music, and ceremonies with profound significance guide and comfort the dying and bereaved.

Spirituality, a broad overarching construct, refers to a personal investment in transcendent values and practices, either within or outside organized religion. Considered "the heart and soul" of religion (Pargament, 2011), spirituality can also be experienced outside religious involvement through personal faith, contemplative practices, humanistic values, nature, the arts, and/or social activism. Spirituality is inherently relational and at the heart of family bonds, from the miracle of birth to life's end and through continuing bonds with the deceased.

Spirituality, seen as a dimension of human experience, expands a systemic perspective to encompass biopsychosocial–spiritual influences and their interplay in personal and relational suffering, healing, and resilience (Walsh, 2009d). Like culture or ethnicity, spirituality involves streams of experience that flow through all aspects of life, from multigenerational heritage to shared family belief systems and their expression in ongoing transactions, spiritual practices, and responses to adversity.

With neurobiological linkages, spirituality involves profound and genuine connection within the self, which is thought of as our inner spirit, center of being, soul, or vital essence. In many languages, the word for "spirit" and "breath" is the same. We are "inspired"—breathing in significant influences; and we "aspire"—breathing out our best hopes and dreams. At life's end, we "expire"—releasing our last breath, which many believe releases the spirit into the beyond. Spirituality also transcends the self, fostering a sense of meaning, wholeness, harmony, and interconnection with all others—from intimate bonds, to extended kin, social networks, and communities, to all life, nature, and the universe.

Spiritual beliefs may constrain or facilitate positive adaptation in facing death and loss (Wright & Bell, 2021). They address the very meaning of life and death and the mystery of afterlife. They provide comfort, hope, support, and connection through the darkest times. They also influence how people communicate about their pain and their preferred pathways in healing. Some who seek help for physical, emotional, or relational problems related to bereavement are also in spiritual distress. Therefore, it is crucial to address the spiritual dimension as a possible source of suffering as well as a potential resource for healing and resilience.

Spiritual Diversity and Complexity

Over recent decades, with growing diversity in societies and families, approaches to spiritual life have become increasingly independent and varied (Pew Research Center, 2015). Adults less often follow the faith traditions they were raised in, shaping their own meaningful spiritual paths within and outside formal religion. Couples and families tend to choose and combine spiritual beliefs and practices that fit their complex lives. Therefore, clinicians should not assume that clients follow the tenets of their stated faith orientation or that the nonreligious have no spiritual connections, concerns, or needs.

Religious affiliation and congregational involvement have been steadily declining among Americans. Yet, the vast majority believe in a Higher Power and in an afterlife, with varied conceptions of both (Pew Research Center, 2015). Over one in four persons describe themselves as "spiritual but not religious." Smaller numbers are atheists and agnostics (who don't believe in, or are uncertain about, the existence of God). Most nonreligious value a broader spirituality or secular humanist values in guiding their actions and relationships. Many turn to Eastern wisdom traditions and meditative practices to nourish their lives.

Spirituality involves dynamic processes that ebb and flow, changing in meaning and significance over the life course. Middle to later life is commonly a time of growing saliency of spirituality, as adults increasingly face the death of loved ones and confront their own mortality. One widower, who had never been "a churchgoer," found that reading Bible passages, especially the Psalms, every evening eased his grief and loneliness. Online religious services, message boards, and spiritual communities offer many ways for isolated or infirm bereaved to benefit from faith-based resources.

Meaningful funeral and memorial observances honor the deceased, comfort the dying and bereaved, and guide them through the most painful life passage. They connect the bereaved with their extended kin and community and transcend a particular tragedy and suffering in their shared human experience. In the Jewish tradition, it is said that grief presents the opportunity to heal and grow through the pain of loss, as expressed in the following Jewish mourners' prayer:

> At times, the pain of separation seems more than we can bear; but love and understanding can help us pass through the darkness toward the light. And in truth, grief is a great teacher, when it sends us back to serve and bless the living. . . . Thus, even when they are gone, the departed are with us, moving us to live as, in their higher moments, they themselves wished to live. We remember them now; they live in our hearts; they are an abiding blessing. (Central Conference of American Rabbis, 1992)

People of many faiths pray for miracles to save a loved one from death, which can lead to a spiritual crisis when prayers are not answered. For some, a profound spiritual experience in threatened death dramatically alters their lives. Many believe that God intends for them to seek greater purpose in life out of a painful loss. Some find solace in the belief that death and loss are part of God's plan and greater wisdom, beyond human comprehension.

Many people find spiritual nourishment and renewal through connectedness with nature or in the expressive arts, inspirational texts, and music. Meaning and purpose are found in generosity and compassionate service or social activism to prevent the suffering of others, to right injustice, or to improve global conditions. Studies find that, in turn, such purposeful actions facilitate their own healing and positive growth.

Contentious social issues such as reproductive rights and assisted dying, while finding growing public acceptance, are strongly opposed among religious conservatives. Yet, we should not assume that individuals or families follow all doctrines of their faith. Intense conflicts can arise around personal considerations in end-of-life decision making or in terminating a pregnancy (see Chapters 4 and 7).

The Mystery of Death and Afterlife

A story is told about a Buddhist novice who asks his teacher what happens after death. He replies, "I do not know." The student, perplexed, queries: "How can that be? You are a Zen master!" His teacher replies: "Yes, but I'm not a dead Zen master."

Belief in passage to a spiritual afterlife has been a core conviction in most religious systems since ancient times—for some, a spiritual realm for eternity and for others, in reincarnation. Buddhist teachings about death focus on spiritual advice to the living: In accepting death, we discover life, able to live more fully and with greater awareness of choices to make the most of our life situations and relationships. Buddhism encourages the dying and loved ones to relate with warmth and caring to what is really happening rather than struggling against it or fleeing in fear. Telling the dying the truth gives them the opportunity to put affairs in order, say their good-byes, and repair past hurts or injustices. Although difficult, it can spur loved ones to communicate caring, love, and trust, without lies or platitudes. Relating in this way conveys a shared acknowledgment that death is approaching, and it encourages those who are important to be fully present throughout this time. Despite leaving partners, family, friends, and communities, the continuity of significant relationships is unbroken by death. Conveying love and connection offers tremendous inspiration to the dying person and to survivors (Nhat Hahn, 2002). Whatever our clients' beliefs and preferences, life's end offers gifts when it is faced with courage and compassion (see Chapter 4).

In many ancient cultures, death and rebirth have been considered essential elements in the never-ending cycle of life. Hindus and Buddhists believe in karma, a natural chain of cause and effect, with one's future lives determined by good or bad deeds in past and present lives. In reincarnation, the soul or spirit may be reborn and inhabit other bodies (or life forms) in successive lifetimes on earth, eventually experiencing spiritual attainment on the path of enlightenment. Native American tribal religions approach death with sadness but without fear, viewing human beings as an integral part of the natural world: death is a transitional event in a much larger life cycle and cosmic unity (Deloria, 1994). As their souls enter the spirit world, their bodies, buried, nourish the plants and animals which, in turn, feed people during their lifetime.

Christianity and Islam teach that at death, the virtuous will find eternal grace, relief from suffering, and reunion with loved ones and ancestors, in an eternal spiritual realm (heaven or paradise). Many Christians, especially African Americans, speak of passing as "going home." The quality of their afterlife will depend on their conduct on earth and their spiritual state at the time of death, with hell and eternal damnation awaiting those who have violated moral precepts. Muslims believe that knowing death is near gives one time to make peace with loved ones, repay debts, and prepare to die. For Jews, it is considered even more important to attend a funeral than a wedding because it both honors a life and marks its loss. Beliefs about a spiritual afterlife are more speculative, with focus on legacies through descendants, achievements, and deeds, especially in actions to repair and improve the world (Tikkun Olam).

Medical science cannot tell us what, if anything, lies beyond death. Clinicians are often reticent to broach the subject. We might simply ask individuals and their loved ones: "What do you believe happens at death?" or "What are your beliefs about the mystery of afterlife?" We can explore their convictions, which commonly ease passage and provide solace to survivors, such as expectations of joining deceased loved ones and ancestors.

The spiritual dimension of death and loss for children is often unappreciated. Even those too young to fully comprehend death may pray for a critically ill grandparent, parent, sibling, or pet, and at death imagine them going to heaven. Well-intentioned attempts to protect children from the sad reality of death can lead to more anxiety, confusion, and upset, as in the following case:

> Richard consulted the therapist for help with his 3- and 5-year-old sons, 2 months after their mother's death. Although the boys had been aware that she was ill and had visited her in the hospital, he had not wanted to upset them, so he didn't tell them she had died or take them to the funeral. Instead, he took them weekly to the cemetery to visit her grave, where, he told them, she was sleeping peacefully. As winter approached, the boys were anxious about their mother's well-being in the cold ground. Richard was at a loss how to help them understand her death.
>
> The therapist explored Richard's faith beliefs concerning what happens after death. Richard said that, as a Catholic, he believed in heaven and pictured his wife there, pain free and serene after her cancer ordeal. The therapist asked if the boys might have any image of heaven. He brightened, noting that they pictured a heavenly place where Jesus lived with God and where angels looked down to protect them. He realized how he could help his boys in facing their mother's death and thinking of her guiding spirit.
>
> Often, when the spiritual dimension is opened in therapeutic conversation, clients handle difficult situations with surprising wisdom and clarity. That evening, Richard told his sons with great tenderness about their mother's death and that she was no longer in pain and was now at peace in heaven. The boys were sad that she wouldn't be coming back, yet relieved to know she wouldn't suffer any more. They talked about heaven, that beautiful place where she would be with Jesus and the angels and would watch over them through their lives. He assured them that they could still take flowers occasionally to her grave to honor and remember her.

Addressing Existential Concerns of Secular Persons

Many people facing death who do not believe in an afterlife still grapple with profound questions about the meaning of life and reflect on their own personal and relational conduct and legacies (Yalom, 2009). Some are troubled by the finality of death and about failing to complete their life work or repair ruptured bonds. Many have larger concerns about the world that will be left to future generations. These might be seen as spiritual matters; yet it's important to respect the preference of many secular persons not to think of their concerns as spiritual, often from their associations with religiosity.

In working with agnostics or atheists, it is important to respect their doubts or nonbelief in God or an afterlife and to ask about their views of a good death and their end-of-life wishes. In a large study (Smith-Stoner, 2007), most atheists reported strong preference for both evidence-based medical interventions and physician–assisted dying and did not want health or pastoral professionals to offer religious prayers or make references to God. They expressed a deep desire to find meaning in their lives, to maintain connection with family and friends, and to deepen connectedness with the natural world through the dying experience.

In therapeutic conversations, it can be helpful to expand our thinking about "afterlife" in terms of the meaning and legacies that one's life will continue to have for others after death. One woman pondered, "Increasingly, I've worried where I will go in people's imaginations. Will anyone remember me? Will I matter to anyone after I am dead?" We can help clients consider the positive legacies they want to leave and take steps, in the time they have, to act on those intentions.

Faith differences in couples should be explored where they create conflict or distance between partners at life's end.

> Scott, age 55, who was dying, kept reiterating his firm scientific conviction that there was nothing beyond physical death and disparaging his wife Val's fervent beliefs in heaven. Deeply pained, she withdrew from him. I asked to hear more about their perspectives in facing death and loss. Scott revealed his own anguish: "I only know my life is over and I'm losing you and all I hold precious." Val reached out to take his hand and replied, "I can't bear losing you, either—that's why I hold onto my beliefs because I don't want your death to be so final." They comforted each other in their grief, as she understood his pain and he realized how her convictions expressed her loving wishes for continuing spiritual connection and reunion.

Recently, a friend who firmly believes in the finality of death shared with me his young grandson's query: "Poppa—where will you go when you die?" Without pondering the complexities, he replied simply, "Into your memories." He added: "So let's make more memories together!," greatly pleasing the boy.

Near-Death Experiences

Near-death experiences (NDEs) are profound phenomena that occur for some persons, both religious and secular, usually in extreme life-threatening episodes, such as cardiac arrest or massive bodily trauma (Koch, 2020). Most common elements include a vivid out-of-body experience, floating above one's physical form and able to see it and its surroundings; often a life review in a "flash"; and passage (sometimes guided by a deceased relative or revered religious figure) toward a bright light or another realm—yet returning to life without reaching it. Many survivors report being profoundly transformed—less anxious about death and more spiritually oriented, with a deep sense of moral clarity and interconnectedness—from interpersonal bonds to larger humanity.

NDEs have been described throughout history, varying in detail with life situation, faith, and culture. Neuroscience explanations attribute the experience to hallucinations produced by brain activity; yet such associations are not necessarily causal, and they are not well understood. They are underreported due to widespread disbelief, ridicule, or pathologizing response, leaving persons feeling unacknowledged, so it is important for clinicians to respect their meaningful experience.

ADDRESSING SPIRITUAL SOURCES OF DISTRESS

In some cases, spiritual beliefs contribute to deep suffering and can block healing. Faith beliefs commonly arise about the cause of a death; it may be seen as misfortune or God's will, or it may be injustice or punishment for transgressions. Spiritual distress may arise with unexpected intensity with death, dying, and loss, even for those who viewed religion as unimportant in their lives. Some may ruminate about their sins or misconduct, worrying about their fate. Families that uphold religious traditions may expect that for one to have a "good" death and a spiritual afterlife, all prescribed rituals must be followed, such as proper burial or cremation (see Chapter 4). Parents who had earlier accepted a child's religious nonobservance, conversion, or interfaith marriage may be tormented by concerns that they (or a grandchild) will not be protected from harm in life or will not go to heaven at death.

Increasingly, medical advances and life support technology are posing agonizing moral and religious dilemmas in end-of-life decision making (see Chapter 4). Some grapple with religious prohibitions about hastening death; many believe it is up to God's will. Such matters can be highly contentious and fuel relational cutoffs, especially if they are not discussed and planned. Sensitive family meetings can facilitate sharing and respect for members' differing convictions and address their anguish and grief.

Moral or Religious Failings, Sin, and Punishment

Concerns about violating moral codes or religious precepts may fuel guilt, shame, or unworthiness and contribute to addictions, social isolation, or suicide. The concept of moral injury, from studies of combat-related atrocities (see Chapter 11), has important clinical relevance. One couple was on the brink of divorce after their child's death. When asked about their faith beliefs, the husband shared for the first time his guilt-laden conviction that this was God's punishment for having killed a child when driving drunk as a teenager. His uncle had "gotten him off" from conviction and told him to just forget about it. His family, relieved, never brought it up again. Referral to a pastoral counselor helped him address his spiritual distress as the couple therapy addressed their shared grief.

Dilemmas in Interfaith Couples and Families

The rise in cross-cultural and interfaith marriages and the growing faith independence from childhood upbringing add complexity to family dynamics with death and loss (Walsh, 2010). With intense emotions at these times, couple or intergenerational religious differences can fuel tensions, conflict, and cutoffs. Tolerance can erode if one faith conviction is upheld as right, true, or morally superior. Therapists can be helpful by encouraging mutual understanding and respect for varied spiritual pathways as well as shared spiritual experiences around common core values.

Even when a client's presenting problems do not ostensibly involve spirituality, a religious concern may become apparent as the therapist asks about their faith. In the following case, religious differences that earlier were unimportant became salient with a tragic loss.

> One young mother, Anna, was referred for therapy by her mother-in-law, who was concerned about her inconsolable grief many months after the stillbirth of her second child. She had withdrawn from her husband, Saul, and was taking their 4-year-old son daily to the grave.
>
> I met with Anna to explore her distress. In asking about the couple's faith orientation, she said she had been raised a devout Catholic but had left her faith in college years. Saul had not followed his family's observant Judaism. Deeply in love, and with religion unimportant to either of them, they had married in a civil ceremony. They had decided not to bring up their first child in either faith and to let him choose his

own spiritual path as he grew older—a common practice in interfaith marriages. However, Anna revealed, the stillbirth of their second child struck her "like a thunderbolt" as God's punishment for not having baptized her firstborn. She had not told her husband or in-laws of her religious turmoil, fearing their upset and rejection. She withdrew in her grief and self-condemnation.

Individual and couple sessions were combined to foster open communication and shared consideration of their spiritual path ahead as a family. Saul was understanding of Anna's religious concerns and assured her of his loving support if she decided to return to her faith (which she eventually did). It was also important for him to be supportive of Anna in sensitively handling what to share about their situation with his worried parents. Consultation with a pastoral counselor who worked with interfaith couples was helpful as they grappled with decisions about religious upbringing for their son and for any future children.

Religious Condemnation, Nonacceptance

Historically, suicide was morally condemned by Jewish, Christian, and Islamic religions, in part to curtail the impulse to martyrdom. For instance, in Catholic dogma, suicide was codified as a mortal sin, burial in consecrated grounds was prohibited, and the deceased's soul was condemned to hell. Such strong theological positions have contributed to stigma, guilt, and isolation for many bereaved families (see Chapter 10). In recent decades, many faith denominations have eased their restrictions, in recognition of the common role of struggles with mental illness or addiction. Because of the staunch religious opposition to assisted dying by persons seeking dignity and control at life's end, advocates urge its distinction from suicide (see Chapter 4).

Heterosexist orthodoxy in conservative religious doctrine has been a source of deep anguish for lesbian, gay, bisexual, queer, and other gender or sexual variant (LGBTQI+) persons in both their couple and family bonds. Some denominations profess a loving acceptance of gay and gender-variant persons but condemn same-sex practices and oppose gay marriage and parenting. This dualistic position ("love the sinner but hate the sin") perpetuates stigma, shame, and a deep schism in gender identity and sexual orientation. Painful issues may arise around denial of hospital visitation, funeral rites, and burial wishes. Parental value systems also impact family acceptance and support, with greater nonacceptance or outright rejection among those upholding conservative religious or cultural views. While many have felt exiled from their childhood faith, most seek spiritual connections in more personal expression and in more inclusive faith communities and chosen family bonds.

Sense of Injustice

The death of "a good person" or an "innocent child" is commonly viewed as unjust and can affect both the spiritual life and relational bonds of the bereaved. Some draw closer to their faith, whereas others question it or turn away. It is important for clinicians to explore varied reactions with sensitivity. Deep anguish can precipitate a family or marital crisis, as in the following case:

> Darla and Greg were referred for grief counseling after their first baby died shortly after birth. The couple and their extended kinship network were devastated. Since the wedding, they had all greatly anticipated this birth—the first son of the first son in a Greek Orthodox family. I asked the couple if their faith was some comfort to them. Darla nodded, saying that the pastor and congregation were very supportive. She now went alone, daily, to church since her husband refused to go. Greg, sitting at a distance from her, pounded his fist on the coffee table, shouting, "I want no more of the church! I'm too angry at God!"
>
> I wanted to understand his strong response. Greg sobbed, "I believe that when something happens there's always a reason. And I just can't fathom what the reason is here. We did everything right, by the book. I don't blame the doctors or the hospital. God took our son! And it's unjust—I don't mean for myself, but to my son. He never had a chance at life. How could a loving God take the life of an innocent baby?!"
>
> Darla said she continued to believe in God's goodness. Unable to tolerate her abiding conviction, he withdrew from her at the very time they most needed mutual support. I recommended a consultation with the hospital chaplain, which helped address the husband's deep spiritual crisis. We focused on their relational issues in couple therapy, aiming to strengthen mutual support in their tragic loss. I encouraged the couple's intention to plan a small memorial service and burial with their extended family. Honoring the birth, death, and loss was healing for all and helped Greg find consolation, support, and renewal in his faith.

SPIRITUAL BELIEFS IN HEALING AND RESILIENCE

Abundant research documents the benefits for health, healing, and resilience by positive spiritual beliefs and practices lived out in daily life, relationships and service to others (Koenig, 2012; Walsh, 2009d). Studies suggest that what matters most is being able to give meaning to a precarious situation, having faith that there is some greater purpose or force at work, and finding solace and strength in these outlooks.

Belief systems are at the heart of coping, adaptation, and resilience in facing death and loss, as discussed in Chapter 2. Spiritual beliefs can foster a coherent worldview and a sense of control (Pargament, 2011). They offer meaning beyond comprehension and render unexpected events less threatening and easier to bear. A grandmother, consoling the family after the death of a grandchild, found her faith supportive: "It's tragic that her life was cut so short, but I trust that God has a bigger picture for us. We'll need to figure out what that is."

Spiritual beliefs can support a positive outlook, active efforts, and perseverance through prolonged suffering or hardship. Hope is essentially a faith-based belief, no matter how bleak the present situation or immediate prospects. Like oxygen for the spirit, hope counters despair and fuels best efforts in overcoming challenges. Faith can support the strength to accept death and loss beyond control. Spiritual moorings can steady the bereaved through turbulent changes. Deep conviction in support by a loving God can bolster courage. One widowed mother, raising three small children, was asked how she finds strength to carry on. She replied: "I talk to God every day!"

A transcendent value system enables members to view their own painful situation from a broader perspective, reducing their suffering and despair. Seeing their struggles as part of the human condition can strengthen their sense of connectedness and common humanity. Spirituality can catalyze positive transformation and growth from suffering and struggle. Some describe an epiphany or awakening to the importance of loved ones, healing old wounds, and reordering priorities. Lives may open to a deeper spiritual dimension, gratitude, and meaningful pursuits. A heightened sense of purpose, generosity, and compassion inspires advocacy on behalf of others for social justice or for the environment (Lietz, 2011).

As bereavement specialists concur, adaptive mourning processes involve the transformation of the relationship from physical presence to continuing bonds through spiritual connections. These can be facilitated through rituals, memories, legacies, deeds, and stories that are passed on across the generations. It can be helpful to encourage later visits to the grave or other meaningful places to reconnect spiritually with loved ones. One woman took her fiancé to her father's graveside for his blessing to marry her. Planting a tree or a garden in remembrance yields new life with the seasons. In traveling around the world, I've found it meaningful to visit a cathedral or place of worship and to light a candle or incense in memory of my mother, a deeply spiritual person who respected all faiths.

Spiritual beliefs can sustain family and community resilience in widespread losses with major disasters and in wartorn regions. In one example, our family therapy training collaborative with mental health professionals in Kosovo provided a resilience-oriented family approach for recovery in the aftermath of the ethnic cleansing campaign waged by Christian Serbs against Muslim Albanians (see Chapter 11). The deep Islamic faith of families and their spiritual connection with the deceased were wellsprings for their recovery and resilience (Becker, Sargent, & Rolland, 2000).

> In one family, the husband, two sons, and two grandsons were murdered in the yard of their farmhouse. The consulting family therapy team talked with the mother and her surviving family members about what kept them strong. The son told them, "We are all believers. One of the strengths in our family is from Allah. . . . Having something to believe has helped very much."
>
> The consultant asked, "What do you do to keep faith strong?" He replied, "I see my mother as the 'spring of strength' . . . to see someone who has lost five family members—it gives us strength. We must think about the future and what we can accomplish. . . . If [my nephew] sees me strong, he will be strong . . . when he [grows up and is] independent, and helps the family—for him, it will be like seeing his father, grandfather, and uncles alive again (Becker et al., 2000, p. 29).

The paradox of resilience is that the worst of times can bring out the best in the human spirit. It often sparks a reordering of life priorities. Spiritual beliefs and practices strengthen the ability to endure and transcend loss and suffering, which, in turn, can lead to spiritual growth.

PRINCIPLES FOR INTEGRATING SPIRITUALITY IN THERAPY

In sensitive inquiry, we explore how clients, from their own distinct sociocultural background, blend the core principles of their faith, or their secular humanistic values, with varied aspects of their lives. For many, traditional beliefs and practices can be a positive sustaining resource in weathering crises. For others, they do not support psychosocial and spiritual well-being. For some, violating core tenets can produce deep internal and relational conflict or alienation. Many seek out alternate constructions and practices within or outside religious structures, consonant with transcendent spiritual beliefs and ethical values without rejecting spirituality altogether.

In clinical assessment, we should not presume that spiritual matters are unimportant if they are not voiced. Therapists who are not religious may underestimate the importance of clients' spiritual beliefs and practices.

When clients are not asked about the spiritual dimension of their end-of-life or loss experience, they may not mention it. The practice guidelines in Table 3.1 are useful to explore (1) the importance of religion/spirituality, (2) spiritual/existential concerns related to death and loss, and (3) potential spiritual resources in healing and resilience.

Clinicians are encouraged to link with pastoral professionals for referral and collaboration on spiritual matters beyond their role or expertise and attuned to their clients' spiritual preferences. It's also good to be knowledgeable about welcoming and inclusive faith congregations and other resources in the community.

All professionals are cautioned to avoid faith-based interpretations or homilies. Others' attempts to cheer or console those suffering by reminding them to count their blessings can trivialize their experience. While well-intentioned, they may not be felt as empathic or helpful when their pain and difficulties are not understood and validated.

When secular clients are struggling with bereavement challenges, some questions to open conversation might be "How do you find nourishment, meaning, and connection in your life and important relationships?"; "When depleted, what resources might replenish your energies

---

TABLE 3.1. Exploring the Spiritual Dimension with End-of-Life and Bereavement Challenges: Sources of Distress and Resources in Healing and Resilience

1. *Explore the importance of religion/spirituality.* Ask about clients' faith orientation:
   • Convey a broadly inclusive perspective of spirituality, including multifaith and nonreligious approaches to spiritual life
   • How meaningful are personal/family faith, spiritual practices, and/or congregational involvement in clients' lives and relationships? In facing death/dying/loss?

2. *Explore any spiritual concerns* that contribute to suffering or relational distress with death/loss and constrain adaptive strivings:
   • Have death/loss wounded the spirit? Sense of injustice (e.g., death of child); alienation from faith; spiritual void
   • Distress or conflict regarding end-of-life decisions, last rites, faith differences
   • Concerns about sin, punishment, or damnation; condemnation of suicide or gender identity/sexual orientation
   • Existential matters: finality of death; life's meaning, purpose; personal/relational harms or regrets; legacy for the future

3. *Identify spiritual resources* (religious and secular) fitting clients' values that might be drawn on to ease distress, find nourishment, and support healing and resilience:
   • Personal faith; contemplative practices (prayer, meditation); rituals
   • Belief in Higher Power, afterlife
   • Faith community involvement; clergy guidance; congregational support
   • Connectedness with nature; expressive arts
   • Social activism to help others, honor memory of the deceased

and bonds?"; "When going through these hard times, how do you find strength and courage?"; "What beliefs and practices could bolster your best efforts?" For those who are not religious, a broader or more personal approach that has greater meaning, purpose, harmony, connection, and fulfillment can be valuable.

In addressing spiritual matters in relational distress, it can be helpful to (1) facilitate communication, understanding, and mutual respect between partners/among family members around religious/spiritual concerns or conflicts; and (2) facilitate compassion and possibilities for relational repair, tapping clients' core spiritual values to support efforts.

PRACTICING A CULTURAL AND SPIRITUAL PLURALISM

A broadly inclusive perspective on culture and spirituality is vital when working with loss, given the diverse and complex beliefs and practices in societies and families today. Despite differences in faith orientation and approaches to death and loss, the overarching aim of spirituality is to be open to the transcendent dimension of life and all relationships, both in everyday practice and in adversity. By practicing a cultural and spiritual pluralism, therapists respect the dignity, worth, and potential of all clients and support their journey in loss and bereavement: seeking greater meaning, connection, and renewal as they move forward in their lives.

Every wisdom tradition, including secular humanism, helps us grapple with universal questions in facing death and loss, such as "Where have we come from, why are we here, and where are we going?" Buddhism counsels us to assume a beginner's mind. As therapists, we most wisely approach the spiritual and cultural dimensions of clients' lives, not from a position of expertise, but by opening our purview to understand their meaning and significance in our clients' lives and relationships.

In working with all clients, it is crucial not to make assumptions about beliefs and practices based on cultural or religious identification or family upbringing. Since many people are increasingly independent in their spiritual life, some may turn to mental health professionals rather than clergy or faith-based counselors, who, they worry, might judge them for nonobservance of tenets. If therapist and clients are of the same cultural or faith background, it may be easier to form a rapport, but caution is needed not to overidentify or to assume shared beliefs. The most important consideration is to hold a nonjudgmental position and understand clients' lived experience, concerns, and salient beliefs and practices.

Many people who come for help with end-of-life and bereavement suffering are seeking more than symptom reduction; many are searching for deeper meaning and connection, a yearning brought to the fore by death and loss. It is most important is to be fully present with those who are dying and those who are bereaved, and to help them tap wellsprings for solace and strength within themselves, in their relationships, and in nourishing cultural and spiritual connections.

Healing and resilience involve a gathering of resources within the person, the family, and the community. Medical interventions may fail to save a life, but therapeutic efforts can foster psychosocial–spiritual healing at life's end and for the bereaved. Therapy best fosters this healing impact by activating relational, cultural, and spiritual lifelines for the relief of suffering, meaningful connection, and renewal of life passage.

Inescapably, therapeutic work involves the interaction of therapists' and clients' cultural and spiritual value systems. Therefore, it is important for clinicians to increase awareness of our own beliefs and family influences and be mindful not to impose them on clients (see Chapter 12). We deepen our therapeutic relationship and effectiveness when we open our work to the cultural and spiritual dimensions of our clients' experience, address their concerns, and tap wellsprings of inspiration to live and love fully in facing death and in living beyond loss.

PART II

Death, Dying, and Loss

Individual, Couple, and Family Challenges

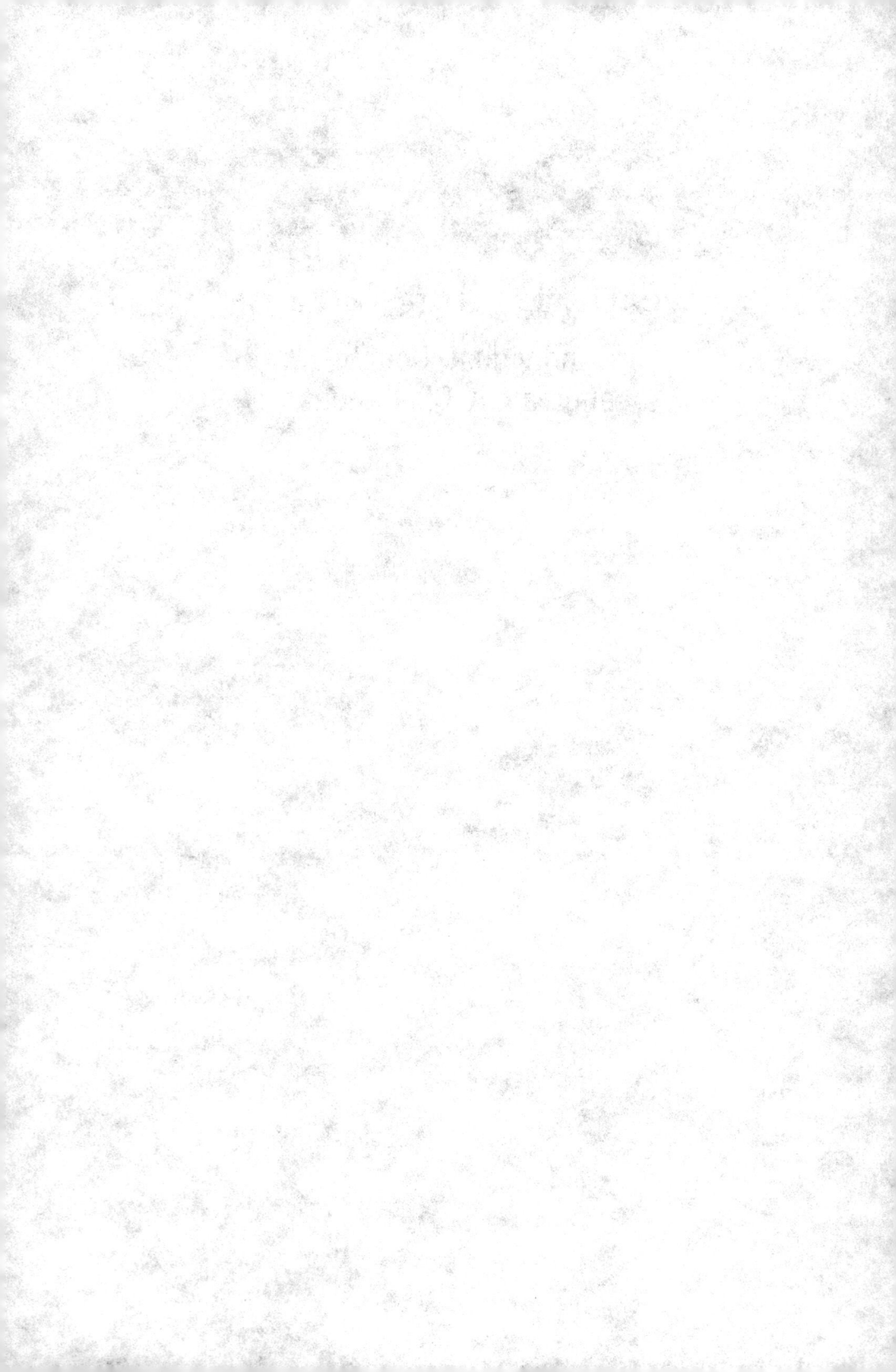

CHAPTER 4

Approaching the End of Life

Challenges and Resilience

> Life changes fast. Life changes in the instant. The ordinary
> instant. You sit down to dinner and life as you know it ends.
> —JOAN DIDION, *The Year of Magical Thinking*

When my widowed father turned 70, feeling lucky for his reasonably good health, he cheerfully repeated one of his favorite adages, "When your number's up, your number's up!" At 74, hospitalized with difficulty swallowing, he was diagnosed with an untreatable esophageal cancer. At first, he mustered up grim humor and fatalistic acceptance that his number finally came up. His luck ran out. Then, learning that he might have just several months to a year to live, my dad erupted in anger, furiously shouting, "They should take me now! Just get it over with!" Yet, in a few days he asked me pleadingly, "Isn't there *anything* they can do? Nothing? I don't want to die!"

My heart went out to him. My love could not save my father's life. I was also overwhelmed with the myriad demands families face. It was complicated: I was his only child, living halfway across the country, with a husband, an infant daughter, and a full-time academic position (see Chapter 12). There is rarely a good time for death to arrive.

For resilience, I needed to practice the art of the possible: to do all I could, in the time we had, to be there for him, meet the challenges, and make the most of precious time. The next 2 months were intense and challenging, yet the most deeply loving time in our relationship.

WHAT IS A "GOOD DEATH"?

Coming to terms with death and loss is the most profound challenge we face in life. Our beliefs about a good death influence our approach to end-of-life challenges, and they can ease or complicate the experience of loss. I've asked clients, students, and colleagues what they would consider a good death for themselves. One friend replied, "No death is a good death!" Yet, considering the inevitability of our mortality, several responses are immediate: "Without pain or suffering"; "Dying peacefully in my sleep"; "At home in my bed"; "Surrounded by loved ones"; "After saying good-byes"; "With time to put affairs in order—but not too much time to be sad." Unfortunately, such idealized scenarios are not the experience in most cases.

As medical advances have prolonged life with chronic conditions, deaths most commonly occur after lengthy and painful struggles with illness and disability. For many, however, death is sudden, without warning or preparation, as with a massive heart attack, or in traumatic circumstances, such as a car crash. Loved ones may not be able to be physically present at life's end, especially those living at a distance. Only one-third of all Americans make end-of-life plans: advance medical directives, funeral planning, and wills or trusts. That leaves most families faced with a cascade of stressful challenges at the most painful time of death and loss.

ANTICIPATING LOSS WITH LIFE-THREATENING CONDITIONS

Life-threatening or life-limiting conditions, as with terminal illness, pose the challenge of carrying on with life in the face of an uncertain prognosis and anticipation of death and loss (Rolland, 2018). Coming to terms with a likely fatal condition is never a once-and-for-all matter but a gradual process over time.

After a diagnosis of breast cancer at age 44, the poet Audre Lorde wrote in her journal, "I carry tattooed upon my heart a list of names of women who did not survive, and there is always a space left for one more, my own." She was a Black, lesbian, single mother with no savings or partner to care for her. She had to work at a job throughout her treatment and was advised to never let on that she was ill. She wrote that, above all, her cancer was a captive fear that she would die and leave her daughter in a hard world with no resources (Lorde, 2020).

Proud at reaching the milestone of 50, Lorde learned the cancer had metastasized to her liver and that surgery would not likely extend her life. She turned to holistic treatments, which improved her quality of life. To make the most of whatever time she might have ahead, she invested in the areas in her life where she could be most effective. She forged resilience alongside anxiety and sorrow: As she traveled and gave lectures, she also sought secret places to cry. Still, Lorde found meaning in doing good work: "I am saving my life by using my life in the service of what must be done." She found joy in mentoring students: "I look at them and they make my heart sing." Above all, she wrote, "I'm proud of having seen my daughter this far. It's a relief to know that no matter how little time I have ahead, she is essentially on her way in the world" (Gay, 2020, p. 101).

A life-threatening illness poses many daunting challenges. Dilemmas may include whether and how long to pursue more aggressive treatments with little or no chance of prolonging life and toxic side effects impairing quality of life for the remaining time. With illness progression and decline, caregiving can become exhausting, financial resources may be depleted, and the needs of a spouse or caregiver and other family members are on hold. Clinicians need to explore the impact on their lives and relational bonds (Rolland, 2018). Loved ones often hesitate to acknowledge their own unmet needs or suffering: "How can I complain when my spouse (or my parent or child) is dying?" It's helpful to normalize the common wish for relief with a death, as it can be guilt-laden for survivors, to respond with compassion for their emotional and practical strains, and to help them find respite and replenishment amid the demands.

THE POWER OF BELIEF SYSTEMS

Our personal and shared belief systems are at the heart of psychosocial healing and resilience when facing death and loss (Wright & Bell, 2021). In couples and families, shared beliefs and practices in meaning making, a positive outlook, and transcendence are key relational processes supporting resilience (see Chapter 2).

Meaning Making

Efforts in making meaning with a life-threatening condition or a dire prognosis support adaptation for affected persons and their loved ones. It is useful to ask what information they have received and what each one believes about the future course, exploring their best hopes and their fears. When medical specialists differ in treatment recommendations, it amplifies anxieties and potential conflict about options. Clinicians can be supportive allies for patients and families in obtaining clearer information about the medical prognosis, treatments, and management issues to guide their decision making. As prospects worsen, we can help them to reevaluate their options and encourage them to focus on ways to master the possible and to accept what may be beyond their control.

Reorienting Hope

In helping individuals and their loved ones living with potentially fatal conditions, it is important not to undermine their hope. We can support their best efforts for optimal chances and quality of life. As an illness progresses, sensitivity is needed to help them reconstruct the meaning of realistic or reasonable hope (Weingarten, 2010). In confronting a greater *probability* of death and as death becomes more imminent, they can be encouraged to reorient hope, prayers, and efforts to ameliorate pain and suffering, enhance comfort, emotional, and relational well-being, and find spiritual peace of mind.

Feelings of despair—literally, loss of hope—can arise when a condition is incurable, suffering is unbearable, or treatment becomes overwhelming. In a couple or family, individuals may be divided in holding onto hope or giving it up (Flaskas, 2007). Therapists need to allow space in the therapeutic conversation to discuss feelings of hopelessness, what hope means to each person, and to support clients in reorienting their vision of hope and mastery to what is possible.

Living with Uncertainty: Holding a Measure of Hope

Helping patients and families live with uncertainty is crucial with a life-threatening condition. The certainty of a fatal outcome or the length of time one may live can vary, depending on affordable and accessible healthcare resources, their overall state of health, and the slow or rapid progression of a condition. With sensitivity and care in timing, we might ask, "What is it like for you to live with such uncertainty?"; "While we all hope for the best, *what if* or *when* things get worse?"; "What would be the hardest parts for you?"; "Who might be most affected?"; "How might your lives change?"; "If a crisis were to end life suddenly and unexpectedly, what regrets might you have about things left unsaid, unasked, undone?"; "Without giving up hope, how might you consider and prepare for the possibility of loss?"; "What might you want to say or do with and for each other?"

Paul Kalanithi, a 36-year-old neurosurgeon, understood his bleak prognosis when he was diagnosed with lung cancer (Kalanithi, 2014, 2016). As a physician, when he had to tell a patient his same age of a dire prediction, he could only muster a few clichés: "It's a marathon, not a sprint, so get your daily rest," and "Illness can drive a family apart or bring it together—be aware of each other's needs and find extra support." Having suspected he might have cancer, he felt a certain relief when he received his diagnosis. Initially, his next steps were clear to him: "Prepare to die. Cry. Tell my wife that she should remarry and refinance the mortgage. Write overdue letters to dear friends. Yes, there were lots of things I had meant to do in life, but sometimes this happens."

In his meaning-making efforts, his wife could not stop his intense reading. "Poring over studies, I kept trying to find the one that would tell me when my number would be up." The large general studies estimated that 70–80% of lung cancer patients would die within 2 years. "They did not allow for much hope. But then again, most of those patients were older and heavy smokers. Where was the study of nonsmoking 36-year-old neurosurgeons? Maybe my youth and health mattered? Or maybe my disease was found so late, had spread so far, and I was already so far gone that I was worse off."

Friends and family members offered anecdotes of someone they knew with the same kind of cancer who went on living for many years. He wondered, wryly, if all the stories referred to the same person, connected through the proverbial six degrees. The path forward would seem obvious, if only he knew how long he had left.

> Tell me three months, I'd just spend time with family. Tell me one year, I'd have a plan (write that book). Give me 10 years, I'd get back to treating diseases. The simple truth that you live one day at a time didn't help: What was I supposed to do with that day? I began to realize that coming face to face with my own mortality, in a sense, had changed both nothing and everything. Before my cancer was diagnosed, I knew that someday I would die, but I didn't know when. After the diagnosis, I knew that someday I would die, but I didn't know when. But now I knew it acutely. The problem wasn't really a scientific one. The fact of death is unsettling. Yet there is no other way to live. (Kalanithi, 2016, p. 95)

Kalanithi advises that what patients seek most is existential authenticity, which they must find on their own. Getting too deep into statistics is like trying to quench a thirst with salty water. The angst of facing mortality has no remedy in probability. He learned a few basic rules for clinicians: Be honest about the prognosis but leave some room for hope. Be vague but accurate: "days to a few weeks," "weeks to a few months," "months to a few years," or longer. He cautioned against relying on detailed statistics, often outdated or acontextual, or googling survival numbers, because we can't predict with certainty for any individual. Mostly, he felt the impulse to keep a measure of hope.

Practicing the Art of the Possible

We cannot control what happens to us, but we can control how we perceive it and how we respond, seizing possibilities, accepting what is beyond control, and living with uncertainty. Jane Brody, the former *New York Times* health columnist, described her own and other women's challenges with cancer recurrence and worsening prognosis (Brody, 2020). They had to learn to accept their limits and to grieve losses—of a professional practice, of their stamina, of the ability to multitask—before they could embrace what remained. She described their resilient responses as a life choice: rolling with the punches, adapting to changing circumstances, and making the best of the here and now, while tackling the logistics of the looming loss in advance.

Brody found that good things came out of the experience, such as gratitude for each day and healing relationships that developed *because* of the illness. She advised focusing more on what is physically, emotionally, and socially possible *now* instead of lamenting what once was and may never be again: "Yearning for a *back to normal* . . . is like a knife to the heart." Instead, she advised creating the best "new normal for now," making life the best it can be each day. Reflecting on her struggle with cancer, Professor Susan Gubar expressed similar thoughts:

> Some find that the darkness of the future heightens the brightness of the present. If this might be the last time I will travel or see my closest friends, I will relish the experience to its fullest. . . . If the next project might not be finished, I will pursue it just as I see fit. Holding a double consciousness becomes a vertiginous high-wire act. It can be debilitating and can be liberating. (Gubar, 2019)

Transcendent Values and Spirituality

In facing the end of life, spiritual matters commonly arise. Therapists are often uncertain about how to broach religious/spiritual issues. Yet, just as we explore varied cultural influences, it is important to include the spiritual dimension of the end-of-life experience, to understand any sources of distress, and to draw on spiritual resources fitting client preferences. To open conversation we might ask, "What are your beliefs about what happens at death?"; "Are there any religious or spiritual concerns that contribute to your suffering?"; "Are religious or (nonreligious) spiritual resources helpful in coping with your situation?" We might encourage our clients to tap spiritual resources, as fitting their preferences, that might be supportive. Since deep spiritual distress is beyond a therapist's expertise, consultation or collaboration with pastoral professionals is advised. With secular clients, it may be important to address concerns about the meaning and significance of their lives and the finality of death. (See Chapter 3 for a fuller discussion and practice guidelines.)

Strong faith can support the ability to meet end-of-life challenges and accept what is beyond comprehension or control. Belief in God or a Higher Power, meditative practices, inspirational texts and music, and congregational support can sustain the dying and the bereaved. Beliefs in an afterlife can bring solace in passage to a heavenly realm and reunion with loved ones, in joining the spirits of ancestors, or in reincarnation to another life on earth. Yet, others may worry that unrepented-for sins will lead to eternal damnation. Some who suffer an unjust or stigmatized loss turn away from their faith. Nonreligious persons may struggle with existential concerns about the meaning of their lives.

Families who are religious commonly expect that to experience a "good" death and spiritual afterlife, traditional rituals must be followed, such as last rites and burial or cremation. Such matters can be highly contentious and fuel relational cutoffs, especially if end-of-life decisions are not discussed and planned in advance. This is a common dilemma in interfaith marriages, as in the following situation:

Rachel, who was Jewish, faced unexpected challenges when her beloved husband, now hospitalized, was close to death. An Ethiopian immigrant, he had long ago left his family's Eastern Orthodox Christian faith and lived by secular humanist values. As he was dying, his only desire was for a simple funeral and burial where his wife could one day join him at his side.

His two brothers, who had been estranged for many years, suddenly appeared at their house, insisting to Rachel that he must have last rites conducted by their priest or he would go to hell. Rachel knew that he did not share those convictions and had to challenge their strong pressure on his behalf. In our consultation session, I encouraged her to invite the brothers to their home for tea and to share stories and photos of her husband's life to know him better and to understand how he strived to uphold the highest moral values in all he did. She showed them awards he received for his community work and photos with their children, reflecting his loving attentiveness as a husband and father. The brothers, genuinely moved, ceased pressing their convictions and were able to share their loving good-byes with him.

To honor her husband's wishes, Rachel sought out the chaplain at the college where they had met, who had known them as students. Now retired, he was honored to conduct a memorial service in the interfaith chapel. Arranging burial was more challenging. Rachel was shocked to learn that only Jews could be buried in the Jewish cemetery near their home. However, they referred her to another cemetery across town with an interfaith site. She found it comforting and knew that her husband would be pleased, that the arch over the entrance to the lovely hillside setting bore the words *Beit Olam*—with the same meaning in Hebrew and in his native Amharic: "at home in the world."

Those who are not religious often lead deeply spiritual lives; many are guided by secular humanist values. Transcendent meaning and interconnection are often found through nature. One mother, seeing her two teenage sons distance from her as her cancer progressed, had a deep desire to take them camping in the mountains. "I wanted them to experience our deep connectedness in nature and to learn that when things get hard, our love, their inner strengths, and their bond as brothers, will support them through life." Her sons, who had not been keen to do the trip, later held the experience as their most precious memory.

Finding Purpose and Meaningful Pursuits

Many studies find that meaningful endeavors that benefit others' lives support resilience in facing death and loss and can leave valuable legacies for survivors.

> Marla, a 44-year-old mother, was feeling stuck, helpless, and hopeless about her terminal condition. Her therapist encouraged her to start organizing family photos and memorabilia to pass on to her children—and to grandchildren she hoped for but wouldn't get to know. That prompted her to begin writing a memoir of her life. She joked, "I know I existed before I was so ill. But as my condition worsened, it has loomed so large in our lives; my kids only know the mom who had cancer—I want them to know my whole life story and learn about our family. And it's a way I can accompany them into their future after I'm gone."

Many find meaning in activism for prevention and treatment to benefit others. One couple, living with the husband's rapidly advancing multiple sclerosis, found a shared sense of purpose by taking part in a research study. They found it helpful that it addressed not only the patient's illness experience, but also that of the caregiving spouse, and the impact for their relationship and their family. He added, "I'm not happy to have MS, but if we can help others, it gives us both deep satisfaction."

In another family, as the father succumbed to the ravages of amyotrophic lateral sclerosis (ALS), his husband and their two children became strong advocates for research and treatment. Clinicians can help families find pride, dignity, and purpose from their darkest times through altruistic actions such as contributions to research and prevention or initiatives to support other patients and families facing similar challenges.

ADDRESSING FAMILY CHALLENGES

Life-threatening conditions have wide-ranging impact for all members of a patient's family, generating emotional turmoil and relational distress. The Family Systems–Illness model developed by Rolland (2018) offers a useful practice framework for positive adaptation. The collaborative approach addresses common practical, emotional, and interpersonal demands with illness progression over time and intertwined with individual and family life course priorities. Therapists encourage families' flexibility to meet emerging challenges over the uncertain course of the condition. It's important to support their efforts to pace themselves to avoid burnout, rebalance relationship and caregiving skews, and juggle the competing needs and priorities of all family members. They may need help to revise individual and shared goals, to adapt to disability constraints, and to sustain intimacy. Families do well by shifting their views of mastery and control over the outcome to making the most of their situation.

When grievances have ruptured family relationships, life-and-death decisions become more complicated. If one adult child becomes overburdened, resentment can brew toward others on the sidelines. Yet, a medical crisis can become an opportunity to heal strained relationships and collaborate as a caregiving team (Walsh, 2016c).

Joleen, a 38-year-old single parent, had an agonizing dilemma. Her father, in a medical crisis, had asked her to donate a kidney to save his life. As a dutiful daughter and a compassionate woman, she felt a sense of obligation: She did not want her father to die because she had denied him her kidney. As we explored her complicated feelings, she tearfully described her father's past alcohol abuse. He had not been there for her as a father and had been a mean drunk. She was enraged to be asked to give up something so vital—what if her children needed a kidney some day?

I broadened the dilemma to include Joleen's siblings, suggesting that she discuss it with them. But she dismissed that idea, saying they had been estranged over the years and were rarely in contact. So, I encouraged her to discuss it with her mother—who then informed her that their father had also asked her brothers for a kidney donation. She was furious, with old rivalries stirred up: who would be seen as the good, caring child or the bad, selfish one? Fired up, she now took the initiative to get her siblings together. When the meeting proved hard to schedule, I supported her persistence. When they met up on Zoom, old rivalries began to melt as they grappled with the shared dilemma.

I expanded their discussion focus forward, wondering if they had considered that other challenges would likely arise in caring for *both* aging parents and for the surviving spouse if widowed. As is common in families, they had avoided looking ahead. I encouraged them to begin brainstorming about ways to collaborate as a team in the immediate crisis—and in meeting future challenges. With this conversation, the oldest brother, Vic, volunteered to donate his kidney for their father. He said he felt less conflicted, remembering good times with him in earlier years before the problem drinking. The others then stepped up, agreeing to support Vic through the surgery. As the beginning of a new solidarity was forged, they agreed to keep in contact and come together around their parents' future needs. Over time, Vic shared stories of their father's life struggles, expanding his younger siblings' understanding and compassion for him.

Although the past cannot be changed, we can help family members expand their perspective and build collaboration and mutual support to chart a better future course. With a terminal condition and a limited or uncertain time to live, members benefit by refocusing priorities, by making the most of the present, and by not postponing important things. A health crisis can spark a sense of urgency. Indeed, couples and families often report that threatened loss brought them closer together, regardless of the outcome. Acknowledging the precariousness of life and the possibility of loss can heighten appreciation of loved ones and can open hearts and minds in relationships taken for granted or blocked by grievances.

Therapists can strongly encourage persons at heightened risk of dying to address important issues proactively—to sort through belongings; discuss medical directives, wills, and gifts; and share vital information such as financial accounts and internet access. Even those with good intentions tend to put off sharing information. As one adult son admonished his parents: "Please don't leave a mess!" Even those who are healthy can suffer a life-ending medical crisis. Recently, a friend of mine, in his 70s, called in distress: his brother, who had been in good health, had had a massive stroke and was given a poor prognosis. As his only surviving kin, he needed to take charge, but he had no idea about his brother's affairs or passwords to his accounts.

In another family, the widowed father made an inventory of family possessions to pass on to his adult children, inviting each of them to select keepsakes, taking turns in choices to be fair. Yet, he was deeply hurt when no one wanted the heirloom china. In a brief family consultation, they reassured him that it was not a rejection of him or disrespect to the family, but a matter of different generational lifestyles. Most often, legacies passed on through values, letters, photos, life stories, and family history are more meaningful than money or objects.

Families commonly avoid conversations about future survivorship concerns. Therapists can coach a client on broaching the issues sensitively.

> Josh worried about how either of his elderly parents would manage alone on the family farm if widowed, but he dreaded talking with them about their death. With his therapist's encouragement, he drove out to the farm, and sat down with them at their kitchen table. First, he asked his mother, tentatively, if she had ever thought about what she might do if she were to lose Dad. She replied, "Sure—we've never talked about it—I wouldn't want him to feel bad. I'd sell the farm and move to Texas to be near our grandkids." Her husband replied, "Well, that's the darnedest thing! I've thought a lot about it too, and if your mother wasn't here, *I'd* sell the farm and move to Texas!" This conversation led the couple to sell their farm, which had become increasingly burdensome, and move to Texas, where they flourished in the company and care of their loved ones.

Facilitating Open Communication: Vital Conversations

In person-centered, integrated healthcare, clinicians help individuals and their loved ones grapple with personal and relational concerns (McDaniel, Doherty, & Hepworth, 2013). Gawande (2014) encourages all helping professionals to facilitate vital conversations, exploring four basic questions:

- What is their understanding of their health or condition?
- What are their goals if their health worsens?
- What are their fears?
- What trade-offs are they willing and not willing to make?

Most important are conversations about their priorities as they approach death and loss. Some want to know their probable life expectancy, while others prefer to hold uncertainty. Some prioritize living long enough for a project completion or a special event, such as a wedding or graduation. Others prefer to end pain and suffering and forego further treatments.

Many people are reluctant to ask questions about life prospects, and medical staff are often hesitant to give "bad news" and are unsure about how much to convey and who to tell (King & Quill, 2006). Clinicians can help family members clarify and evaluate differing medical opinions, which increase distress. Often, spouses or family members disagree about the path forward, sparking conflict or distancing. Couple or family sessions can be valuable to share viewpoints, weigh options, and facilitate understanding of differences and decisions reached. Engaging in end-of-life decision making can be emotionally draining, so it is important to pace tough conversations and encourage ways to find respite and moments of enjoyment to revitalize spirits and bonds.

Sensitivity to family belief systems is also important, such as values in some cultures not to plan for death or discuss it openly with the patient (see Chapter 3). Sometimes communication is blocked by anxiety that talking about death may bring it on. Some worry that the patient may think that they want them to die. Some feel guilty in wishing for an end to a long ordeal. It is helpful to explore such concerns, normalizing and contextualizing them as common and understandable in the family's situation.

Children's understanding of death and dying changes as they mature (see Chapter 6). One of the hardest things for families is to tell a child that the parent has a very serious condition and may not survive it.

> Janelle, a single parent, called the mental health clinic after finding her 10-year-old daughter Keisha's letter to her camp counselor saying she wanted to die. Janelle had recently learned that her metastatic cancer was no longer treatable. Trying to be upbeat for her daughter, she kept her busy, avoiding discussion of her terminal condition. Keisha heard her mother crying late at night, but not wanting to burden her, she showed no outward sign of her upset. The therapist encouraged Janelle to share her medical situation, hold her through her distress, and plan activities to share. Keisha asked her mom to teach her how to cook their favorite recipes, which her mom had learned from Keisha's grandmother. While cooking and enjoying their dinners together, Janelle shared stories of growing up in her family.

A youth's maturity, relational connectedness, and empathy are all fostered by encouragement to keep connected to their parents through a fatal illness, death, and loss. It is crucial for parents to encourage them to voice their concerns and to keep the door open as other concerns surface over time.

When children are critically ill, parents often want to shield them from the painful understanding that they will likely die. Yet, children are often aware of their worsening condition, as are their siblings. Some, feeling protective toward their parents, may not want to make them sad by opening a conversation and revealing their own concerns. Recent guidelines for families encourage them to speak openly with children when they or their parent or another important family member faces life-threatening conditions and may not survive (Dalton et al., 2019). When family communication is shut down around the threatened loss, the unspeakable may go underground to surface in other contexts or in a child's symptomatic behavior, as occurred in the following family situation:

> An expert in child sexual abuse consulted me about a puzzling case. A mother had brought in her 4-year-old son, Rico, concerned that he might have been molested at preschool because in recent weeks she kept finding him fondling himself. The evaluation revealed no indication of sexual abuse. To understand if Rico might be expressing anxiety about other concerns, I suggested that she meet with the parents and explore recent stresses in the family. The mother, again coming alone, revealed that 7 months earlier the father had been diagnosed with stomach cancer and had undergone extensive surgery to remove the tumor.
>
> It was important to explore how the family had coped with that life-threatening crisis and its aftermath. Not wanting to worry the children, the parents had minimized the "procedure" and had not mentioned cancer. At her husband's hospital discharge, he had insisted on going "back to normal" and put the incident behind him. To respect his wishes, they told the children, "Daddy is fine now," and they said no more about it. When I asked how this life-threatening experience had affected her, she became tearful, saying that it had shaken her sense of security, but she kept her worries to herself. Then 2 months ago, a suspicious new growth was found in his follow-up, heightening her concerns: he might die, and how would she manage? Not wanting to worry the children, they said nothing to them and assumed they were OK, since they never asked questions about their father's health. After a pause, she noted, "Now that I think about it, one night recently, when saying bedtime prayers, Rico added, 'And please, God, take care of Daddy's tummy.' "

When life-threatening concerns are not voiced, spouses may avoid contact, and children, keenly sensitive to the tense family atmosphere, cope alone with greater anxieties. Clinicians can be helpful in opening blocked communication by facilitating and shaping difficult conversations. In the family above, it was important to meet first with *both* parents, helping them (1) to face together the worsening prognosis, share their concerns, and strengthen mutual support; and (2) to convey information about developments sensitively with their children and support them through emerging challenges. In conversations, they might ask each child what they understood about the situation, what they worried about, what they hoped for, and what would help. Most children benefit from open, honest communication, becoming calmer and less anxious.

It's also important to ask about and respect individual and family preferences as to how much they prefer to share beyond their closest kin. Some value their privacy, whereas others appreciate support from a wide social network. Parents might want to talk about their situation with the parents of their young children's playmates, as anxieties sometimes lead others to avoid contact so their child doesn't worry about dying or losing their own parent.

Social Discomfort and Support: What Hinders, What Helps

Kate Bowler (2018b), a divinity professor living with Stage IV colon cancer, described her painful social interactions: "We all harbor the knowledge, however covertly, that we're going to die, but when it comes to small talk, I am the angel of death. I have seen people try to swallow their own tongue after uttering the simple words 'How are you?' I watch loved ones devolve into stammering good wishes and then devastating looks of pity."

When needs for family and social support are so important, many avoid contact because of the discomfort and awkwardness in not knowing what to say. Contact also confronts others with their own looming fear of losing someone they care about and the acute, terrifying awareness of their own mortality. Social discomfort also contributes to well-intentioned but unhelpful responses. Some minimize the significance of one's experience by making a comparison to worse fates, beginning sentences with "Well, at least. . . . " Others press to keep endlessly cheerful—"You're so strong—you'll beat the odds!"—or offer platitudes, such as "God never gives you more than you can hold."

Instead, it can be helpful to begin with acknowledgment, such as simply saying, "I'm so sorry this is happening for you." Hope need not prevent acknowledging losses and hardship. Next comes loving appreciation. Yet, Bowler cautions this should not sound too much like a eulogy; she notes that she's actually had kindly letters written about her in the past tense. The impulse to offer encouragement is valued. For many, there is tremendous power in touch and in thoughtful gifts: seemingly small efforts—a friend drops off cookies and another takes her to a concert—are anchors that hold her to the present. On a very bad day, they remind her, "Yes, the world is changed, but do not be afraid. You are loved. You will not disappear. I am here" (Bowler, 2018b).

Seizing the Moment: Reconnecting and Healing Frayed Bonds

"I got word that my brother died. I knew he had Stage IV cancer—We'd been estranged; I meant to call him, but it never got to the top of the list." Too often, in my practice experience, clients come to therapy after a significant loss, filled with regret and recriminations over ruptured bonds unrepaired, apologies not made or accepted, important questions unasked, or love never expressed. The most bitter tears shed over graves are for loving words unsaid and deeds undone.

Facing death and loss can be an impetus for estranged family members to reconnect and to repair strained relationships before the opportunity is lost. Often, this requires overcoming reluctance to stir up painful emotions or old conflicts. Some may fear that direct confrontations or opening painful issues could increase upset and cause death. In some cases, it would be important to coach the patient and family to consult with their healthcare provider for assurance that heightened emotions would not bring on a medical crisis. It's crucial to deal sensitively with these concerns, interrupt destructive escalations, and help family members to share feelings constructively with the aim of healing pained relationships.

A facilitated *family life review* (Walsh, 2016c) can foster greater understanding and a fuller, evolutionary perspective of family life and relationships. In sharing reminiscences, both the highs and the lows, family members can incorporate varied subjective experiences in their shared life passage. As members recall hopes and dreams, important milestones, and both satisfactions and disappointments, the conversation enlarges the family story, builds mutual empathy, and can heal old wounds. Therapists can help to clarify misunderstandings, to place hurts and disappointments in the context of life challenges, to recover caring aspects of relationships, and to update and renew relationships that have been frozen in past conflict or alienation. With the passing of elders, precious conversations can be recorded and family photos, stories, and genealogy can be shared before personal accounts are lost. Wisdom can be drawn from past hardships, and stories of resilience can inspire survivors' journey ahead.

In seeking reconnection, ways must be found to express hurt, anger, and disappointment and yet with consideration toward others, as the following case illustrates:

Jorge, age 32, had been estranged from his father since leaving home in anger after high school. His father's recent heart attack led his mother to urge Jorge to mend their relationship. She had always tried, unsuccessfully, to smooth over their conflict. Jorge held intense anger from his father's harsh criticism throughout adolescence: Jorge could never please him. Yet he was reluctant to confront him because respect toward elders was a strong value in their culture. Avoiding contact had been his survival strategy. Now, he feared that expressing his anger would ignite his father's explosive reaction, which could be fatal, due to his weak heart.

Yet, not trying would leave his own wound festering after his father died. The therapeutic challenge was to open these sensitive issues in a respectful rather than an attacking way, with the goal of reconciliation.

The father, pained by Jorge's estrangement, was open to family sessions to repair their bond. The therapist encouraged Jorge to think ahead for the meeting and to keep focused on that intention. He might start by affirming his respect for his parents and perhaps by expressing appreciation for something positive in their family life that he was grateful for. At the session, the mother sat close to the father, holding his hand to support him. Jorge thanked his parents for the strong values they had given him. He said he shared their desire to repair the rift. The therapist asked if he might start by sharing any happy memories with his father from his childhood. He smiled as he recalled tossing around a football in the yard, feeling close and laughing together at stupid jokes. He then related how hurtful his teen years were, receiving his father's harsh criticism, feeling unable to please him, and believing he was a disappointment to him. He asked, "Were you ever proud of me?"

The father hung his head, remaining silent. The therapist asked what was going through his thoughts. He said that he had suffered constant berating and humiliation by his own father and had fled from home by immigrating and never saw him again. He now realized he had turned into his father, driving away his son. He added that it was his own sense of failure that led him to push his son so hard. "I didn't know how to show you praise." After a pause, he looked into Jorge's eyes and said, "I'm so sorry for that." Jorge was deeply moved by his father's account and his genuine remorse. After the session, the father sent Jorge a folder he had kept in a desk drawer—he had saved clippings of Jorge's high school and college activities and awards. He enclosed a note, for the first time expressing his pride and love. Jorge visited soon after, expressing his own love and gratitude.

As families approach death and dying, they are often more open and honest about earlier transgressions or shame-laden secrets and more readily acknowledge and regret past ruptures and hurts, opening possibilities for relational repair. Therapists can facilitate fruitful conversations to clarify misunderstandings and faulty assumptions. Earlier conflicts or hurts can be reconsidered from new vantage points. This involves a process of mutual reengagement, with a readiness of each person to take the other(s) seriously, to acknowledge violations to the relationship, and to experience associated pain. More than righting wrongs, a process of reconciliation leads to deeper bonds, mutual understanding, and well-being (Hargrave & Zasowski, 2016). At life's end, the simple words "I'm truly sorry" and "I love you" mean more than ever.

ADDRESSING CHALLENGES NEAR LIFE'S END

Owen, age 45, wished to spare his parents upset—he was their only child—so he did not tell them of his untreatable melanoma until 3 weeks before his death. In the shock of this sudden loss, his father suffered a heart attack and his mother fell apart emotionally. They had had no time to process the diagnosis or its progression over the past year and were filled with regrets about all they would have done differently if only they had known.

Sensitive communication between the dying and the bereaved is vital, as loved ones confront the reality and grapple with its ramifications. Family-focused interventions can prevent complicated bereavement in families with relational and communication difficulties. In a large, randomized, controlled trial, Kissane and colleagues (2016) found that 10-session family-focused therapy during palliative care for advanced cancer and continuing into bereavement reduced the severity of complicated grief and the development of prolonged grief disorder in high-risk families with low communication and in those with high conflict.

Drawing up and discussion of living wills and directives by all adult family members (not only the patient) are most helpful to share important decisions and to reclaim the dying process more actively. It's also crucial to plan and discuss meaningful funeral rites or memorial events, wills, and legacies, honoring the wishes of the dying person. This can avert later conflicts and ease the burdens and misunderstandings of survivors. Authorization of organ donation most often brings solace and meaningful benefit in enabling another life.

It's essential for clinicians to attend to needs for pain control. Family collaboration is important in making arrangements to keep the dying person comfortable and comforted. Family members often most fear witnessing their loved one in uncontrolled pain and can be reassured that for over 90%, good pain management can be achieved without cognitive compromise. Palliative care—which does *not* require treatment termination—reduces pain and suffering and enhances well-being and dignity. Hospice, based on a philosophy for compassionate end-of-life care, tailors services to meet the needs of each dying person and their family members, either in care settings or at home whenever feasible (Caserta, Lund, Ulz, & Tabler, 2016). Hospice professionals offer compassionate psychosocial and spiritual support attuned to patient and family concerns and provide moments of joy and respite through music and other expressive arts. Some persons nearing life's end are turning to an ancient practice, calling on a *death doula*, who provides emotional support through the dying passage.

With racial disparities in healthcare, Black, Indigenous, and Latinx families are less likely to have access to affordable treatments, advance directives, hospice care, and adequate pain management at the end of life. Therapists should sensitively explore structural barriers to care and support their active steps to gain vital information and services. Encouraging open communication among family members is important, as many are reticent to talk about death or plan for it. While most want to pass peacefully at home with loved ones, too many die in emergency hospitalizations, alone and undertreated for pain. There is an urgent need for information, care, and planning—with family involvement—to benefit not only the terminally ill, but all who might die unexpectedly (Rolland, Emanuel, & Torke, 2017).

End-of-Life Dilemmas in Decision Making

We all hope to die peacefully and with dignity. Yet urgent medical crises and biomedical advances increasingly pose anguishing dilemmas concerning whether and when to prolong treatment or end life support measures. They raise a profound question: what is a "natural" death in our times? Families often must make heart-wrenching decisions, which are most agonizing when a death was unanticipated, advance planning was not in place, and disorientation is highest. Such decisions also raise profound questions of when life ends and who should determine that end, involving medical ethics, religious convictions, patient and family rights, and even criminal prosecution.

Family bonds can be torn apart by conflicting views.

> In one close extended family network, Varda, the elder sister and legal healthcare proxy for their mother, made the difficult decision, based on the physician's prognosis, to end life support efforts when the mother's organs were failing and there was no chance of recovery. Her sister accused her of "killing" their mother, the beloved family matriarch: "Only God can decide when it's time to die," she insisted. The sister cut off further contact and would not allow her children to play with their cousins. Varda came for therapy 3 years later, tormented by the death and with an "aching heart" to reconnect with her sister and family.

Family consultations, preferably before a life-or-death crisis, can be valuable to help members share feelings and perspectives about complex situations, allow them to focus more fully on the patient's needs, weigh various options, and come to terms with decisions taken (Rolland et al., 2017).

Medical Aid in Dying

Increasingly, persons with intolerable pain and debilitating, life-limiting health conditions express the strong need for personal agency: to have control and choices in ending their lives. As unbearable as uncontrollable physical suffering is the loss of autonomy, dignity, and quality of life. Both therapeutic and bioethical issues arise, and many physicians are unwilling to consider any assistance in dying. Persons who are most religious tend to oppose any actions to hasten death. Yet, attitudes concerning choice and compassion in end-of-life decisions have been changing, with over 7 in 10 Americans currently supporting the right of terminally ill people to die on their own terms. Death with dignity is increasingly seen as an end-of-life option and a fundamental human right (see *https://www. deathwithdignity.org, https://compassionandchoices.org*). A growing number of states are legalizing this option as ethicists and mental health and health-care associations increasingly adopt policies to support the choice of mentally competent, terminally ill persons to exercise some decision-making control for a peaceful and dignified death. Yet, the issue remains highly controversial, and many are unaware of laws facilitating or constraining end-of-life options.

It's important to clarify terms and distinctions. Unlike *euthanasia*, where the physician plays an active role in dying by injecting a lethal combination of drugs, *medical aid in dying*, or *patient-directed dying*, allows terminally ill, mentally capable adults to request from their doctor a prescription for a lethal dose of medication they can decide, at any time, to self-ingest to die peacefully in their sleep. This affords them control in determining the time and place to end their life, with the opportunity for loved ones to be with them and say their good-byes. Some individuals keep the medication nearby but never use it, reporting that it eases their minds to know they have the option available. Clinicians are advised not to refer to assisted dying as "suicide," which carries the stigma of pathology and mental illness (see Chapter 9) and is inappropriate, disrespectful, and distressing for mentally competent, terminally ill persons. As individuals and families increasingly confront end-of-life decision making, medical, legal, and moral/religious issues all require thoughtful discussion and consideration.

FACE-TO-FACE WITH DYING:
MAKING THE MOST OF PRECIOUS TIME

When the physician Oliver Sacks faced the end of his journey with cancer, he felt a sudden clear focus and perspective:

I cannot pretend I am without fear. But my predominant feeling is one of gratitude. I have loved and been loved; I have been given much and I have given something in return . . . but now I am face-to-face with dying. It is up to me now to choose how to live out the months that remain to me. I have to live in the richest, deepest, most productive way I can . . . Over the last few days, I have been able to see my life as from a great altitude, as a sort of landscape, and with a deepening sense of the connection of all its parts. This does not mean I am finished with life. On the contrary, I feel intensely alive, and I want and hope in the time that remains to deepen my friendships, to say farewell to those I love, to write more, to travel if I have the strength, to achieve new levels of understanding and insight. . . . There is no time for anything inessential. I must focus on myself, my work and my friends. This will involve audacity, clarity and plain speaking; trying to straighten my accounts with the world. But there will be time, too, for some fun. (Sacks, 2015a, 2015b).

For loved ones, even brief interactions near life's end can be profoundly moving exchanges, with tears commingled with laughter and humor.

At the death of her wife, Lori, after a debilitating illness, Mika was sad but also at peace: She shared a diary entry with her therapist. "The simple fact is that Lori's body stopped. There was no unfinished business between us. Yet I had carried a lot of fear about death and I didn't want to go on living without her. Lori showed me how to feel more alive and more open, even in her last days. She accepted that she was dying, even though she didn't want to go. Acceptance didn't mean feeling happy or that she liked the situation, just that this was the truth. I'll always miss her, yet I know I can go on to live and love more fully, carrying her spirit with me."

The end of life may hold unexpected gifts for families when members fully engage with each other and make the most of precious time.

Sean, age 52, came to talk with me about his unbearable sorrow at his mother's terminal illness. We explored his complex feelings. A devout Catholic, she had done all she could to keep her family intact while enduring an abusive marriage and many uprooting relocations due to his father's alcoholism and repeated job loss. After the father's recent death, Sean had bought a new home for his mother in high hopes that, at last, she could enjoy her later years in peace and comfort. He was devastated that her serious condition so quickly shattered these dreams. "It's just not fair! She deserved some good years."

At adulthood, Sean and his sisters had scattered around the country and maintained little contact. Since their mother's cancer had rapidly spread, she had uncharacteristically encouraged them to make several trips to visit and help out. Now she had just called them together, he feared, for their last good-byes. He was tormented as he left for the visit.

When I saw him after his return, Sean seemed transformed: his inner turmoil had subsided. I asked, "So, your mother didn't die?" He replied, "Oh she did die—but *how* she died was amazing!" I asked to hear more. "I knew my mother was a strong woman, but she was most incredible as she faced her own death—I realized she deliberately brought me and my sisters to care for her, time and again, in order to knit us back together. Her final request made sure that we'll continue our bonds. She told us she didn't want to be buried where she lived, far away from her children and her roots. Instead, she asked to be cremated and that we take the urn with her ashes and go together to each town where our family had lived and scatter some of her ashes in a beautiful place we had enjoyed. Her love and courage inspired us to honor her wishes even better. We told her we would save a portion and make a trip to Ireland together to scatter the last remains in the town of her grandparents, where she had always wanted to visit. She was so pleased and died peacefully a few hours later as we sat around her singing Irish ballads she had loved."

This potential for personal and relational transformation, forged through suffering and loss, distinguishes the concept of resilience from coping and surviving. As we've seen, resilience in facing the terminal illness and death of a loved one involves more than shouldering pain or a caregiving burden and bearing the sadness of all that is lost. Sean's moving story reveals the core of relational resilience: Family members rallied together to practice the art of the possible. They made the most of limited time and transcended the immediate death and loss, inspired by their mother to carry out her wishes, thereby honoring and sustaining her memory and spirit. In the process, their lives and bonds were enriched. In resilience-oriented practice, we can strive to facilitate both healing and transcendence.

CHAPTER 5

In the Wake of Loss

Fostering Healing and Resilience

Grieving allows us to heal,
to remember with love rather than pain.
—RACHEL NAOMI REMEN

In the aftermath of loss, surviving loved ones navigate varied pathways in grieving and moving forward with life. In systemic practice, therapists attend to the loss experience and foster healing and resilience—which are understood as human capacities involving family, community, and larger sociocultural resources. Greater attention to grief in the family context is needed (Breen et al., 2019). Death poses the most painful and far-reaching challenges in family systems, and family processes are central in positive adaptation.

FAMILY ADAPTATIONAL CHALLENGES WITH LOSS

While there is wide variation in modes of dealing with death and loss, families confront common adaptational challenges. How they respond can complicate grief and adaptation, or they can support healing and resilience for all members and their bonds.

In developing a systemic approach to loss, grounded in clinical research, Monica McGoldrick and I identified four major family tasks that influence immediate and long-term adaptation (Walsh & McGoldrick, 1991, 2004). (Worden, 2018, described similar tasks for bereaved individuals, based on his early study.) We view these as relational processes that families actively engage in and clinicians can facilitate. They involve an interweaving of key processes for resilience in the three domains of family functioning: belief systems, organizational patterns, and communication/problem solving, as outlined in Chapter 2.

Acknowledging the Loss: Rituals and Social Support

Family members, each in their own way, need to confront the reality of a death and to grapple with its meaning and implications for themselves, for other members and their bonds, and for the family unit. With the shock of a sudden death, this process may start abruptly. As discussed in Chapter 4, contact before death offers the opportunity for each member to express their love and say their good-byes. Well-intentioned attempts to protect children or vulnerable members from contact to spare them potential upset can isolate them, stir anxious fantasies, and impede their grief process.

In the immediate wake of loss, clear and open communication facilitates grief processes. Yet clinicians must be mindful of individual, family, and cultural differences in norms and preferences for sharing information and emotions (see Chapter 3). It's most important to support a climate of trust, respect for varied perspectives, and empathic responses of family members to each other. Sharing clear information about the facts and circumstances of the death, while painful, helps members absorb the reality of the loss. One who is unable to accept the reality may avoid contact or become angry with those who are grieving. When a death and loss are faced courageously among loved ones, relationships can be enriched.

Rituals marking the end of a life have been central in all cultures and religions over time (Walsh, 2009c; see Chapter 3). Across faiths, funeral rites and memorial services provide direct confrontation with the reality of death, the opportunity to pay last respects, and a way for the bereaved to share grief and receive comfort with extended kin and community (Imber-Black, 2012). Increasingly, loved ones actively participate in memorial events—through meaningful eulogies, personal stories, and artistic expression—to remember and celebrate the person, their life passage, and important relationships. In one moving tribute to their father, a daughter from his second marriage recounted poignant and humorous anecdotes from her childhood; then his son from a former marriage, saying he was never comfortable with words, played a stirring flute melody he had composed in his father's memory.

In New Orleans, the jazz funeral cortege is a powerfully transcendent rite to mourn and honor the deceased. Dating from the late 1800s and the birth of jazz, the ritual embraces both tradition and generational change, with bands now mixing in funk and hip-hop (Fausset, 2019). Following the religious church service, community members gather, a mix of cultures, races, and ages, some in Mardi Gras attire. They follow the band accompanying the hearse on the deceased's last trip through neighborhood streets. The cortege is also a celebration of rebirth: Slow dirges give way to joyous, up-tempo beats and cathartic dancing as the body releases the soul, ascending to heaven. Mourners cry out, "God, she went home"; "Fly away, baby. Fly away."

Sharing the experience of loss, in accord with personal beliefs and preferences, is crucial in the healing process. Whether through conventional or innovative memorial tributes, clinicians can encourage family members and social networks to plan gatherings. Internet live streaming now enables remote participation for those unable to attend in person. Social network postings of death announcements, increasingly common, can be meaningful if done thoughtfully. One daughter of immigrant parents created a website for extended kin and friends near and far, on which she had composed a moving tribute to her father, begun in the months before his death. She shared stories and photos of his life journey and important milestones in their family life. Visitors to the site shared remembrances; some renewed valued contact with dear ones long out of touch.

Drawing family members together on an anniversary or at a holiday gathering to remember one who has died can be a healing and connecting experience. Therapists can facilitate their conversations to open possibilities:

> One father consulted me with concern about his 15-year-old daughter, Tania, who had refused to attend her mother's funeral at her death a year earlier and was still withdrawn from the family. As I explored the family's loss experience, I noted that the approaching Mother's Day might be especially hard for them. Yet, it could also be an opportunity for a small, meaningful remembrance. I suggested that he invite Tania and her brother, Derek, to help him plan a loving way to remember their mom, rather than making arrangements himself, as he had done for the funeral, and then trying to coax them to show up. First, it would be important to acknowledge with them the sadness Mother's Day would likely arouse, and then all the more important on that day to share their loving remembrances. Derek suggested they meet up with their grandparents on the riverfront at sunset. Tania objected, emphasizing that it would be too sad to watch the sun go down. Moments later, she flashed a smile of inspiration: "Let's meet there at *sunrise,* when mom loved to take the dogs. She would love that!" Their shared experience, commingling deep sadness and treasured memories, opened Tania's blocked grieving and fostered mutually supportive bonds in their healing process ahead.

Open Communication: Facilitating Grief and Meaning-Making Processes

The complexity of bereavement in couples and families can be challenging, considering individual members' varied impact and reactions. Communication processes are vital in sharing the emotional pain of grief and providing mutual support. As a family experiences a loss, members touched in varied ways may show a wide range and fluctuation of responses, depending on such variables as their age and individual coping styles, the state of their relationships, and different positions in the family. Members' tolerance for varied reactions and timing is important when they are out of sync. Strong emotions may surface at different moments, even months later, including mixed feelings of anger, disappointment, helplessness, relief, guilt, or abandonment, which are common to some extent in most relationships. In some families and cultures, the expression of intense emotions can generate discomfort and distancing by others. Moreover, fears of loss of control in sharing overwhelming feelings can block all communication about the loss experience to protect oneself and each other.

Therapists, particularly when working with an individual client, need to explore the varied reactions and their interplay in couples and in family systems (see Chapter 1). When grief is blocked or distorted in families, emotions often explode in conflict with others, particularly in couple, parent–child, sibling, or extended family bonds. One member may internalize their grief in symptoms of anxiety or depression, while another externalizes distress in problematic behavior. Some try to escape unbearable pain through alcohol or drug use. If a family is unable to tolerate certain feelings, a member who directly expresses the unacceptable may be scapegoated or frozen out. In a relational system, overwhelming emotions may be expressed in fragmented ways by various individuals: One may carry all the sadness, while another is in touch only with anger; one may show only relief, while another is numb. The shock and pain of a traumatic loss can shatter family cohesion, leaving members isolated and unsupported in their grief (see Chapter 9).

Shared meaning-making processes are crucial for adaptation. They involve narrative attempts to put the loss into some meaningful perspective that fits coherently into a family's belief system and life experience. This includes the ongoing negative implications, especially the loss of future hopes and dreams. Nadeau's (1997, 2008) qualitative research explored family meaning-making processes with the death of a family member. In interviews with nonclinical, multigenerational bereaved families, she found that the story of "what happened" emerged from a process of co-construction. Families employed many approaches, including storytelling, dream sharing, comparing the death to other deaths, "coinciding" (attaching meaning to events that occurred near the time of the death), and characterizing qualities of the member who died. Families also engaged in "family speak," weaving together individuals' threads of meaning. Their communication patterns included agreeing/disagreeing, referencing other members' meanings, and cooperative interrupting by supporting, echoing, finishing sentences, elaborating, and questioning. Family meaning-making was sometimes facilitated by the participation of in-laws who, less susceptible to family rules, could open discussion of taboo subjects. Problem solving at the family level involved finding solutions to instrumental issues, such as interactions aimed at filling the vacant role in family functioning. Nadeau's study revealed the ongoing interplay of beliefs, organizational patterns, and communication.

Reorganizing Family Functioning

The death of a family member leaves a hole in the fabric of family life. It disrupts established patterns of interaction. The process of adaptation involves a realignment of relationships and redistribution of role functions to compensate for the loss and to carry on. Often, family reorganizational demands must be addressed before parents or caregivers are able to deal with their own grief. Extended family involvement can help surviving family members reorganize daily patterns of living and provide appropriate care for children and vulnerable members through the disruption.

> Family life was upended for Alex, 33, and Daria, 31, and their three small children, ages 6 years, 4 years, and 18 months, when Daria was diagnosed with leukemia. The couple had to travel a long distance for bone marrow replacement, and several inpatient stays were required over the following months. After initially rallying, Daria died at year's end. Both extended families came together in support throughout the lengthy ordeal. Two aunts took turns doing "homestays" with the children, providing loving care and minimizing the disruption in their lives. Other relatives offered their emotional and practical support to relieve strains. After Alex returned to his full job responsibilities, their families pitched in financially to hire a housekeeper/caregiver for the children to bolster family efforts. Over the years, the Aunties continued to play a prominent role for the children and in family life.

Without support, family role responsibilities can interfere with grief. The demands of jobs, needed income, and child or elder care may constrain parents' emotional expression. Children may suppress their own needs to bolster a bereaved parent or caregiver whom everyone depends on, particularly in multistressed, single-parent families. Therapists need to help families structure the time and space for grieving, needed respite from demands, and ongoing family functioning. It's useful to ask about daily and weekly routines, what has changed since the loss, what is most stressful, and what would help. Resilience is fostered by encouraging members to rally as a collaborative resource team, so all can play a part and no one is overburdened. Community services are vital for support.

It is important to help families pace their reorganization. If a family takes flight from losses by moving precipitously from their homes or communities, further dislocations will generate more disruptions and loss of social supports and local resources. Children must adjust to new surroundings, a new school and peers, and the loss of friends, teachers, or mentors and valued activities. Some individuals seek immediate replacement for their losses through new intimate relationships or affairs, sudden marriages, or pregnancies. These replacement relationships run the risk of complication when loss and grief are unattended (see Chapter 10).

At the other extreme, some families hold on too rigidly to former patterns in living that are no longer functional, as in the following case:

> After her husband's death, Maureen vowed to carry on family life and to raise their two daughters according to his standards. She took a stressful job to pay bills, yet she continued to keep the house spotless and prepare the father's favorite meals, keeping his empty chair at the head of the table. She came for therapy 4 years later for help with conflict with two of her daughters, now in adolescence, over her insistence on continuing family traditions they had outgrown. In a family session, they expressed their desire to spend more time with friends and to give up elaborate meals and activities they only pretended to enjoy. Yet they didn't want to be disloyal. Maureen acknowledged her exhaustion in straining to be "two parents" and live up to her husband's idealized values. We worked on finding ways to honor the father's memory, sustain valued continuities, and yet make needed changes in their structure as a single-parent family to reduce strains on the mother and to better fit the daughters' emerging developmental priorities.

Family structures can crumble with an overwhelming loss. Leadership and communication may falter, and parents may be unable to nurture and protect children. As we saw in Hope's painful experience (see Chapter 1), children can suffer not only from a parental loss and exclusion from family mourning processes, but even more by further separations, confusion, and lack of protection in the aftermath of loss. It is important to provide clear information about what they expect to happen, when, and who will take care of them. With the death of a parent, it is natural for children to worry about losing the surviving parent or other caregivers. Reassurance and trust that they will be nurtured and protected are vital. Every effort should be made to keep siblings together, as their bonds can be essential lifelines.

Social supports often dwindle after the first few weeks of a loss, so it is crucial to link those who are bereaved and isolated with kin and community support over the many months that follow. Adaptational challenges can pile up in the first year. In our culture's ethos of self-sufficiency and aversion to depending on others, people often are reluctant to ask for help. Encouraging them to think of ways for mutual exchange, or future intentions for paying back or paying forward, can promote a healthy relational interdependence for resilience.

Reinvesting in Other Relationships and Life Pursuits

As time passes, survivors need to reconfigure their lives and relationships to move forward, reenvisioning life aspirations. For many, relationships taken for granted become more valued. For others, a loss prompts them to leave unfulfilling or troubled situations. Often, new and unforeseen life directions open up.

In some cases, the formation of other attachments and commitments can be blocked by idealization of the deceased, a sense of disloyalty, or catastrophic fear of another loss. Others may take flight from painful losses through precipitous replacement by a new partner or another child. Well-intentioned friends or relatives may rush a widowed parent unwisely into premature remarriage "for the sake of the children," risking complications if mourning processes were unattended. A bereaved spouse's rapid remarriage can spark upset by children or former in-laws if they view it as disloyal. Often, children balk at accepting a new stepparent when their loss has not yet been attended to or integrated in family life. Therapists can help families to avoid pitfalls in navigating and pacing their steps ahead.

> In working with Maureen and her daughters, I encouraged them to sort through sealed boxes stored away from their past family life, choosing keepsakes and sending mementos to relatives. For the approaching anniversary of the father's death, Maureen decided to write a tribute, which she had been unable to do at the time of the death. This prompted one daughter to write a poem and the other to make a drawing in memory of their father. With enthusiasm, they gathered these mementos together and sent them to relatives and friends, reviving valued contacts that had been lost.

This unpacking and reconnection led Maureen to request couple sessions with her companion Larry. Within a few months of her husband's death, she had plunged into this intimate relationship, and at his urging to start a new life, she had moved with her daughters to his city. But now she felt "stuck" and ambivalent about remarrying. Larry admitted that he, too, needed to think it over. Formerly married, his wife had abruptly left him, and he was skittish about making another full commitment. The following week, he arrived at the couple session near the end of our time. A large man, out of breath from rushing, he plopped down on the sofa, which cracked down the middle and fell apart. Apologizing, he remarked that maybe the sofa forewarned their breakup. Although they cared deeply about each other, they agreed to go their separate ways.

When a significant death and loss have not been mourned and the survivor rushes into a new attachment, the breakup of that replacement relationship can open unexpectedly strong grief from the earlier loss.

In the weeks after her breakup with Larry, Maureen was surprised to start dreaming of her deceased husband for the first time, waking in tears with a deep yearning for him. We met in individual sessions to address her previously unattended grief. I find it helpful to start by remembering the person and their relationship through reminiscences and photos of their life together as it evolved from the beginning over time. She recalled their meeting and dating, and then traced the milestones, joys, and hard times in their marriage and childrearing over the years. A strong regret she still carried was their argument the night before his sudden death in a car crash; she wished she had made up with him before he left in the morning for work. She sobbed, "If I had only known I'd never see him again!"

In the next session, using an "empty chair" technique, I coached her to imagine what she would want to tell him if he were sitting there now. She began by saying how sorry she was for her part in their petty fight. Tears flowed as she conveyed how much she loved him and reminisced about some treasured times: he was the love of her life. We sat in silence for several moments, holding those feelings before ending the session. I asked her if, in the next session, she would like to update him on the developments in family life since his death. In that session, she related their move to start a new life, and how hard it had been for her to shoulder all the financial and childrearing responsibilities without him. Speaking about their daughters, she shared how pleased and proud he would be at how smart and beautiful they had become. I added my praise that she had done a remarkable job on her own.

In the following session, we talked about her guilt-tinged feelings of anger and abandonment at how her husband's death had left her with the "heavy load" she had been shouldering. She said she now felt it was time to ease up on her unrealistic expectations about providing the "perfect family" for her daughters and to expect more of them, in sharing responsibilities to earn their privileges.

At a follow-up session 3 months later, she and her daughters looked happy and more relaxed. Although the girls grumbled at their newly assigned tasks, they enjoyed greater independence and a warmer relationship with their mom. She had found a new job with better hours and benefits and began singing in her church choir, which brought her joy and connection. Those new steps bolstered her resolve to stick with a weight-loss program, losing the physical "overload" she had been carrying.

Our clients' remarkable ingenuity can emerge through our work. In this case, we flexibly combined family, couple, and individual sessions as priorities emerged. When we approached Maureen's spousal grief, she asked me if she could record our sessions. Looking back when we ended our work, she said, "Now that I have it all recorded, I don't need to carry it in my head anymore. I can file it away and listen to it whenever I want to." She understood what she needed to do to unburden herself—mind and body—and regain her spirit to thrive.

PRACTICE PRINCIPLES, PRIORITIES, AND GUIDELINES

A resilience-oriented systemic approach with loss is guided by an understanding of family challenges, variables that heighten risk, and key relational processes that foster coping and positive adaptation. Given the diversity of family forms, values, resources, and life course, we must be careful not to confuse common patterns in response to loss with normative standards or to assume that differences in bereavement are pathological. Helping clients deal with loss requires respect for their beliefs and encouragement to forge their own pathways through mourning and adaptation. Therapy is most successful in helping the bereaved when we bear witness to their loss, suffering, and struggle, and we support their strengths and potential to overcome life challenges to thrive. Table 5.1 summarizes practice principles to foster healing and resilience with a significant loss.

Varied Modalities in Systemic Practice

A systemic framework in practice explores and addresses the reverberations of a death and loss for individuals, their relationships, the couple or

TABLE 5.1. Practice Principles to Foster Healing and Resilience with a Significant Loss

- Collaborative approach with individuals, couples, and families
- Respectful language, framing to humanize and contextualize distress
  - ♦ View as understandable, common in complex or traumatic loss situation
  - ♦ Decrease shame, blame, pathologizing
  - ♦ Offer research-informed understanding of grief processes
- Provide safe haven for sharing pain, fears, and challenges with loss
  - ♦ Compassionate witnessing for suffering and struggle
  - ♦ Encourage loved ones to share experience, meaning making, and mutual support
    - ◊ Facilitate their understanding and respect with varied responses
    - ◊ Address loss-related conflicts; facilitate shared decision making
- Convey conviction in potential to overcome loss-related challenges through active efforts over time
- Identify and affirm strengths, courage alongside vulnerabilities and constraints
- Tap into kin, community, and cultural/spiritual resources
  - ♦ Identify and build individual, couple/family capacities for healing and resilience
  - ♦ Strengthen key processes in family resilience
  - ♦ Mobilize support in social networks/community/larger systems
  - ♦ Tap cultural–spiritual resources
- Shift focus from problems to possibilities; accept what is beyond control
  - ♦ Reorient hope from despair; re-envision future aims and priorities
  - ♦ Support varied pathways through grief in coping, healing, and adaptation
  - ♦ Support learning, change, and growth from the experience
- Integrate experience of loss and resilience into chapters of individual and relational life passages

family unit, and social contexts. We attend to the multiple influences in bereavement throughout the relational network, including important roles and relationships within and beyond households, biological and step relations, and both extended family and informal kinship bonds. Individual, couple, and/or family sessions may be combined flexibly to fit varied loss situations and challenges over time.

In working with individual clients, coaching techniques can facilitate and process their relational conversations or change efforts outside sessions. A spouse, siblings, a caregiving grandparent, or other family members may be involved in brief conjoint sessions. Couple or family sessions are valuable in facilitating important conversations, observing and addressing relational dynamics, and healing relational wounds. Members unable to convene in person and those living at a distance can take part through telehealth conferencing.

Family contact may range from consultation and brief intervention to more intensive therapy. For instance, family meetings are helpful in sharing information or in decision making. Individual or conjoint sessions can be useful to understand and address issues of various members and subsystems (e.g., spousal, sibling, or extended kin) as relevant. Decisions at various points are guided by a systemic view of loss and emerging priorities.

Resilience-oriented groups can be helpful for those confronting similar loss challenges, such as couples who suffered perinatal loss, families bereaved by suicide, and those affected by collective loss experiences, as in disaster or war-related recovery and refugee resettlement. Facilitated groups can provide useful information and participants' sharing of painful experiences, mutual support, and strategies for coping and resilience. Therapists offer compassionate listening to participants' common and unique experiences of loss, affirm their strengths alongside their suffering and struggle, and encourage their active collaboration for adaptation. Bereavement groups can also be valuable in sharing the stories, values, and meanings of the lives of the deceased: remembering them, accessing their voice, and expanding painful memories to include more complex and contextualized perspectives, all aiming to continue connections that are compassionate and empowering (Hedtke, 2012).

This resilience-oriented approach, building on general principles in strength-based systemic practice with individuals, couples, and families, focuses on the impact of a tragic loss in relational systems. It is broadly inclusive of sociocultural, developmental, and multigenerational influences in vulnerability, risk, and resilience. Therapeutic efforts aim to support bereavement processes, build capacities to surmount loss-related challenges, and regain the spirit to thrive.

Assessment Priorities

In bereavement inquiry, we assess family functioning, the state of relationships, and changes with a significant loss. We explore (1) the impact of the death and loss for the family system, its members, and their relationships; and (2) the family approach to the loss situation, including its preparedness, immediate coping responses, and long-term adaptive strategies. Both the factual circumstances of a death and the matrix of meanings it holds in the family need careful exploration.

It's important to focus not only on problematic family patterns but also on positive strengths and potential resources that can contribute to healing and resilience. Therapists might ask about the ways in which a family has dealt with other adversity, highlighting stories of resilience that might inspire efforts to master current bereavement challenges. We search for relational resources in coping and for both practical and emotional support through extended kinship, social, and community networks and in cultural or spiritual resources.

The *genogram* (family system diagram) and timeline can be helpful tools to guide inquiry and visualize complex relational patterns schematically, including significant roles and bonds within and across households; extended kin and social supports; and socioeconomic, racial/ethnic, and other relevant variables (McGoldrick et al., 2020). A timeline is valuable in noting past, recent, or anticipated losses; other significant events or major stressors; and their potential relevance to presenting problems. Even a brief sketch noting key members, bonds, and timing of critical events can be useful. In the following situation of couple conflict, a highly significant past loss was brought to light:

> Vanessa and Marcus sought couple therapy to resolve intense conflict over having a second child, which she very much desired and he vehemently opposed. The initial therapy focus on their current relationship issues and future life visions did not help, as Marcus grew more agitated. Brief family of origin inquiry by the consultant revealed that Marcus's mother had died in childbirth with his younger sibling, a devastating loss he had suppressed and had never shared with anyone. In exploring that experience, with Vanessa's empathic understanding, Marcus realized his catastrophic fear of losing *her* in childbirth: She was the love of his life, and he couldn't bear to go on without her.

Multistressed families, often in low-income, underresourced communities, are especially vulnerable to a pileup of internal and external stressors that can overwhelm functioning, heightening risks for subsequent problems. Extended kin and social support are crucial to enable family members to attend to grief processes and other priorities.

> Brent and Jasmine, parents of three small children, sought counseling on the verge of divorce, with escalating conflict and Brent's heavy drinking. Brent was attending AA and an anger management group. Brief couple therapy focused on reducing emotional reactivity in their interactions, but no family history or contextual influences had been explored.
>
> Invited as a consultant, I asked about their family life and any recent stresses, tracking events over time on a family timeline. Brent choked up, relating the sudden death of his brother 2 years earlier in a car crash. His father, distraught, suffered a massive heart attack and died. Brent had then struggled unsuccessfully to save their small family business. With

their town's economic decline, the business failed, and he found only part-time work. As a result, the family lost essential income and health benefits. Then, the maternal grandmother—their mainstay in raising their young children—suffered a debilitating stroke; and Jasmine, now pregnant, needed to attend to her care as well. The couple was reeling from crisis to crisis, with mounting pressures fueling their distress and conflict. Brent said they were just trying to keep their heads above water and had not focused on their losses or realized their impact.

Resilience-oriented couple counseling helped them to contextualize their current crisis in light of the family's cascade of stressful losses and challenges. Sessions offered them a space to share their grief and facilitated their mutual support, family role reorganization, and team efforts, tapping extended family and community resources.

Exploring Social, Cultural, and Spiritual Influences

Expanding our lens, we explore social, cultural, and spiritual influences that can complicate or support bereavement and positive adaptation (see Chapter 3). We give particular attention to social inequities, discrimination, and barriers for racial/ethnic minorities and other marginalized groups. We explore the role of cultural and family norms and address intergenerational and gender-based constraints in grieving processes.

Because religious/spiritual concerns commonly arise with death, dying, and loss, it's essential to explore clients' faith beliefs and practices (see Chapter 3). We shouldn't presume that spiritual matters are unimportant if they are not voiced or if clients are not religious. Just as we would inquire respectfully about cultural beliefs and practices, we need to show comfort and interest in exploring the spiritual dimension of their loss experience. It's crucial to understand how religious or existential concerns may contribute to suffering and how spiritual resources, fitting our clients' value systems, might be resources in healing and resilience. Consultation with pastoral care professionals can be helpful in addressing a deep spiritual crisis.

THE THERAPEUTIC PROCESS

In our therapeutic work, it's important for clients to feel both permission and safety to open and share deep pain, intense emotions, and confusion with assurance that we will not judge or abandon them in their suffering or worsen it. We offer compassionate witnessing, as well as strong support, encouragement, and perseverance, to overcome the fears and protective barriers that can block mourning and adaptation.

Compassionate Engagement: Stories of Love and Loss; Suffering, Remembering, and Renewal

As clients grapple to make meaning of their loss situation, practitioners' genuine concern is most important. Too often, people in their lives turn away, uncomfortable with strong emotions or uncertain how to respond. We need to listen openheartedly to very painful accounts of all that has happened and to their ongoing struggles. It is most important to convey our assurance that we can bear to hear about their suffering and that we will offer a safe haven for them to contain and process intense emotions. At the same time, we need to notice, ask about, and highlight moments of loving care and sparks of resilience.

One couple came for counseling after the tragic death of their baby, Sophie, just 10 months old. In contrast to common gender-based differences in couples dealing with tragedy, Adam, a Chechen immigrant, was emotionally distraught and requested help for himself; Nora, his American wife, said she was coping well and didn't need therapy. But, at my request, she agreed to come for couple sessions to support Adam.

> Adam began by explaining that he came for therapy because he had suffered terribly in the past, through the brutal war and atrocities in Chechnya, and had fallen into a dark hole in the aftermath. He said that losing his child was even more devastating and he wanted to get help so he wouldn't fall into an even deeper pit. We spent the next few sessions going over the painful events of the past year and all their loving efforts, which he related through tears. After a normal birth, doctors had discovered a rapidly growing brain tumor at a 3-month checkup. They underwent grueling ordeals of surgery, radiation, and chemotherapy but were unable to save Sophie's life. Adam didn't regret all the treatments; he was glad they had done their best. But the loss of her precious little life, after all that, was more than he could bear.
>
> A few weeks later the couple went to visit close relatives in another city. In our next session, Adam was distraught: he was furious at them. After dinner, with no mention of Sophie or their loss, as they sat around over coffee, a cousin quietly muttered that he was sorry for their loss. Adam asked if he would like to see a photo of Sophie and handed it to him. His cousin was so uncomfortable he only mumbled, "Oh, how sad." He quickly passed the photo to the person next to him, who glanced at it, muttered "So sorry," and passed it on. And so it went around the room, awkwardly, until someone changed the subject. The couple left early, feeling totally abandoned and isolated in their grief.
>
> I said I would very much like to see photos of Sophie if they would bring them to the next session. Adam replied, "I have them right here

on my iPhone!" and he eagerly pulled it out. He had taken photos at her birth—and a photo every day in her struggle to live. I pulled my chair up close to the couple.

I expressed my interest in starting with her birth and early hopeful months and hearing about their joyful times. They shared moments of their delight in their newborn and how beautiful she was, how full of life. I held the iPhone with Adam as we scanned through the many photos from the diagnosis through the treatments, tracing their journey. I asked him to pause at photos that stood out and were most meaningful for them and to tell me about those times. I listened intently and shared my observations. In one photo, Sophie lay in a hospital bed, hooked up to tubes and monitors; in another her head was bandaged after surgery. I acknowledged how hard that must have been, pausing as they recalled that experience. I then also noticed how beautiful her eyes were as she gazed directly at her mother, holding the camera. Adam remarked, yes, he thought she was trying to reassure them not to be so worried, that she was pulling through. In one photo, she had lost her hair; I asked if they had saved any of her beautiful curls, and Nora smiled and nodded. In the last photo, Adam was lying in bed, holding tiny Sophie on his chest, his arms encircling her. I commented on his loving embrace and the peaceful smile on her face. I was quiet as Adam and Nora sobbed and held each other for quite some time. As we ended the session, I commented on Sophie's remarkable strength in enduring her painful treatments, and I told them how much I admired them for their loving care of Sophie and their ongoing mutual support through their darkest times.

That session marked a turning point in the couple's healing process. Over the following weeks, Nora started a scrapbook, including favorite photos and Sophie's lock of hair. Adam became more animated, resuming his activities, and returned to his neighborhood soccer games, where teammates welcomed him back.

As in this case, therapists can foster healing by offering compassionate witnessing for clients to "re-member" the fullness of their relationship with their deceased loved one (White, 1989) and to grieve their loss. Our attentiveness, leaning in rather than sitting back, conveys our interest in understanding and validating all that they had gone through. Our nonjudgmental questions and observations give encouragement to explore and express a deep well of feelings without need to consider what they "should" feel or concern about making us uncomfortable.

Fostering Meaning Making of the Loss Experience

In collaborative practice, it's important to learn the subjective perspectives of clients and appreciate their life experience. It's crucial to explore the multiple meanings that loss situations hold and to be mindful not to make assumptions based on our own beliefs or experience. We need to understand their core beliefs and expectations that influence their coping approach and their difficulties in making needed adaptations. It's important to address constraining beliefs, which may be conveyed in pessimism or despair, or in blame, shame, and guilt. We can support more facilitative beliefs for a more hopeful outlook and active agency in surmounting bereavement challenges.

In respectful inquiry, we might start by offering our condolences for the loss, and then ask about the death event. "What happened?"; "I'd like to hear more about your experience." We explore the information they received and their understanding of the nature and circumstances and ask about varied perspectives by family members and any lingering questions or concerns. With sensitivity, we ask about the person and significant relationships lost. We inquire about family role functions and hopes and dreams altered. In exploring the impact, we might ask, "What stood out for you as most upsetting in the loss experience?"; "What are the ripple effects for couple/family members and relationships?"; "What has been most challenging in recovering from the loss?"; "How do you and your loved ones try to cope and adapt?"; "Has anything been remarkable, helpful, or reassuring?"; "Who and what might help now, and how?" Such inquiry acknowledges both the shared and unique experience in families as it explores the subjective views of members and their beliefs on what is most meaningful, troubling, and inspiring.

It's especially important to support families in helping children and vulnerable members to make sense of a death and to provide reassurance that they will be secure and well cared for in the aftermath (see Chapter 6). The bereaved tend to do better when they can understand more fully what happened, how it came about, the future implications, and what steps they can take to cope and adapt. Some may need help in tolerating unclarity about their loss situation or future uncertainty. Resilience is fostered as we help individuals, couples, and families gain a shared sense of coherence, rendering their crisis experience more comprehensible, manageable, and meaningful to address (Antonovsky & Sourani, 1988).

A common challenge for the bereaved is that many aspects of a loss situation may remain unclear. Information about a death may be insufficient, inconsistent, or difficult to comprehend. A death may be senseless. The future may be in flux. It's important to ask clients about their own and their loved ones' understanding of their loss situation: what they experienced, what they have been told by experts or others, and what they each believe to be the case. Family members may hold quite different perceptions or assumptions. As a challenging situation becomes increasingly stressful, relational tensions heat up.

Therapists can encourage clients' efforts to gain and share crucial information to ease anxieties and support active coping. We can assist them in locating reliable community resources and reputable internet sites. We can coach members in navigating larger systems, such as pressing medical or legal professionals to help them sort out complicated or conflicting information about a death. A family consultation can be useful to share information gathered and to plan the next steps.

Humanizing and Contextualizing Distress

In a culture that touts the virtues of self-reliance, those who are struggling are often hesitant to seek help. Concerns about blame, shame, or failure to "get over" their loss contribute to their reluctance to come to therapy and to early dropout. When losses and grief are disenfranchised (i.e., socially unacknowledged and/or stigmatized; see Chapters 7–10), they may expect to be judged negatively or their pain minimized by professionals.

Systemic descriptions that humanize distress facilitate emotional and relational healing. Because the very language of therapy can pathologize individuals and families, we take care in framing problems, questions, and responses in a way that is respectful of distressed individuals, their families, and their situations. We avoid demeaning labels or pejorative language about "dysfunctional families," and we unhook assumptions of pathology and deficits from the rationale for involvement in therapy concerning bereavement challenges. When working with individual clients, we indicate that we might want to suggest inviting a spouse or family members because they may well be affected by the loss and because they could be valued resources or partners in our client's healing process.

A resilience orientation heightens appreciation of all clients' unique experiences and beliefs, as well as commonalities with others facing similar life challenges. The aim is to depathologize, humanize, and contextualize distress. We must be careful not to oversimplify the complexity of loss-related challenges and neither minimize problems nor trivialize an experience of suffering. Every loss should be honored and should not be compared to other, more dire situations.

Therapists can offer new perspectives to help clients see individual symptoms, strained relationships, or a breakdown in family functioning as understandable and/or common in their complicated loss situation. *Reauthoring and reframing* are means to expand a constraining approach to troubling situations through language and perspective, casting a bleak situation in a new light that is more amenable to positive change. When used genuinely and respectfully, therapists can offer a useful new perspective, generate hope, counter a destructive or blaming process, and overcome impasses.

Distress is humanized when it is seen as a common reaction under highly stressful conditions. Traumatic stress reactions are viewed as normal responses to abnormal, traumatic events and experiences. Unhealthy behaviors or withdrawal from a partner might be seen as survival strategies in response to feelings of vulnerability (Scheinkman & Fishbane, 2004), in an attempt to live with an unbearable loss, to prevent a feared outcome, or to signal a need for help. While being cautious never to condone or excuse harmful behavior, we may note benign or helpful intentions behind misguided or hurtful actions. When a painful loss situation can't be changed, bereavement challenges might come to be viewed in more empowering terms that facilitate healing and resilience.

Rekindling Hope amid Tears

While being empathic with the struggles of despairing clients, it's crucial to acknowledge their despair and, with sensitivity, to rekindle their hope. For example, we may say, "I understand that you're experiencing a lot of pain and conflict right now. It is a lot to bear." Reaching for relational support, we might add: "I'm also convinced that you have many strengths, personally, and as a couple or family. I believe that within the turmoil, you care deeply about each other. I'm quite hopeful that with mutual support you can come through this difficult time. I'll be glad to work with you and to support your best efforts as you move forward from darkness to light."

Kaethe Weingarten (2010) offers the idea of *reasonable hope* as a practice, as something we *do*, preferably with others, and aiming toward a goal. Reasonable hope fosters resilience by practicing the art of the possible— seeking realistic goals and pathways rather than those desired but unattainable. We can't bring a deceased loved one back to life and we grieve that loss. Yet, we can transform our attachment from physical presence to continuing bonds sustained through spiritual and symbolic connections that remember and honor our loved one.

When clients have lost hope, we might ask, "Can you recall a time when you felt more hopeful about your situation? What was helpful? Who supported that hope? How?"; "How might you harness that positive energy now?" Conversations can explore what might be learned and applied from past times of adversity to the present loss situation, as well as what could help to regain hope. What might a partner, parents, or others say or do that might comfort. Often, one spouse will turn to the other and say, "I just need you to reassure me that we'll get through this together." A spouse or parent may need to hear that they are valued and that their efforts matter. Small acts of kindness and expressions of gratitude and mutual appreciation can bolster spirits.

Practicing reasonable hope is not the same as blind optimism. We recognize the complexities and contradictions of lives and losses, acknowledging doubt, contradictions, and despair. In going forward, we view the future as open, uncertain, and malleable. With death and loss, hope may need to be reoriented; clients may have to revise goals and seek pathways they never imagined or thought they could accept. The practice of hope can provide a deep spiritual contentment, connecting us to the webs of meaning and relationship that make life purposeful. Those who are hopeless must resist isolation by connecting with others. Those who are witness to despair must resist indifference or numbing out. In couples, when one spouse loses hope, the other can hold it for both.

Practicing the Art of the Possible

For healing and resilience in the wake of loss, therapists need to support active agency in *mastering the possible*, helping clients to focus their efforts on what can be done, accepting what is beyond control and tolerating uncertainty. One of the most difficult challenges is coming to accept a death and loss that cannot be changed. In working with those deeply wounded by bereavement-related struggles, we need to diminish self-blame and shame and foster compassion. Remorse is common for things done or not done in a loss experience, especially under stressful conditions. We can help clients to own regrets and any accountability, and to learn from them for the future.

Many families need help in tolerating future uncertainty. We may need to support efforts to cope with a loss-related precarious situation, such as financial and housing insecurity with the death of a breadwinner. When prospects remain murky, we can encourage efforts to find creative approaches or new life directions.

Steps toward a Positive, Future-Oriented Vision

After a shattering loss, survivors sometimes become stuck in a vision of their lives that is narrow and joyless, filled with yearning, remorse, and fear. Helping clients to reorient their hopes and dreams encourages them to imagine a more satisfying future and take steps toward achieving it. It shifts emphasis from a deficit-skewed focus on all that has been lost to possibilities to reimagine and rebuild lives. Together, we and our clients can then envision possible options that fit their situation and reachable aims through constructive efforts. This effort involves imagination, a hopeful outlook, and initiative in taking actions toward desired goals.

In helping clients move forward, it's important to resist the impulse to simply "put the loss behind" or seek "closure" by locking away the painful experience in a sealed vault. Rather, connections can be made and revisited between the past, present, and future to more fully integrate the experience. We can't change the past, but we can help clients learn and grow from it and gain perspective to chart their future course.

Gaining New Strengths, Insights, and Purpose

As the bereaved begin to move forward in their lives, therapists can support their efforts to gradually integrate their loss experience in the fullness of their life passage and relationships. We encourage them to explore what might be learned from their experience. There may be important lessons about risk and vulnerability. Often, something valuable is gained from a loss experience that might not have been learned or achieved otherwise. Often, it is realization about their own capacities to surmount the worst that can happen: "We now know that we can get through anything life throws at us." Loss of a loved one may bring a heightened recognition of the importance of other relationships that had been taken for granted or written off. A family relocation prompted by loss can also be a milestone, a time to reassess life and relationship priorities. A crisis can lead family members to question, review, and redirect their lives. A woman who had completely oriented her life around her husband felt lost herself when he died: "I didn't even know who I was without him." Therapy facilitated her life transformation from an initial sense of emptiness to the development of new talents and confidence in her own identity and ability to lead a fulfilling life. New pathways to growth can be forged out of shattering loss.

By strengthening key relationships and family functioning, a healing process can reverberate throughout the network to benefit all members. While open communication and mutual support are emphasized, active collaboration in dealing with death and loss are also encouraged, ranging from the drawing up and discussion of wills, living wills, and directives to planning and participating in meaningful memorial events and remembrances over time. In cases where mourning has been blocked, we can encourage clients to sort through old photos and memorabilia, which open memories and trigger the flow of old stories and new reflections. In sharing stories and mementos with children, other family members, and friends, a chain of positive mutual influences is set in motion.

Bereaved families often find strength to surmount heartbreaking loss and go on living a meaningful life by bringing benefit to others from their own tragedy, such as through organ donation, memorial contributions, or compassionate initiatives or community action coalitions. Clinicians can support clients' efforts to find pride, dignity, and purpose through their darkest hours through altruistic actions that honor the life or the best aspirations of the deceased.

Being Fully Present

As therapists working with death and loss, we need to accept our own limitations and understand how we can be helpful. More than one client referred for griefwork has said, "I don't know what good therapy can do—you can't bring back my loved one!" For therapists trained in brief solution-focused approaches, this reality can be especially challenging. Death is not a problem to solve, and the technique of asking the Miracle Question (de Shazer, 1985) would be inappropriate. If the bereaved are asked, "If a miracle were to occur, what would it look like?," many would reply, "That my loved one would still be alive." Jumping quickly over distress can trivialize clients' experience and shut down their grief. Rather, therapists need to be compassionate allies with clients in exploring complex loss situations, encouraging their openness as they grapple with the ramifications in their lives.

What matters most is being fully present with our clients, helping them to tolerate intense emotions and attend to suffering without sinking into despair, helping them to move forward on a healing path. Bereavement and adaptation take time. We may be with them for only a short while on their journey, but we can be at their side, accompanying them on this stretch of the way.

In the following chapters, we'll address the many complex and traumatic loss situations that complicate grieving and adaptation. In all our endeavors to help clients facing the challenges of death and loss, what is perhaps most important is what we, as helping professionals, bring to the therapeutic encounter in our own beliefs, emotions, and experiences concerning death and loss. In Chapter 12, we'll address the challenges of compassion fatigue and explore the therapeutic interface of clinicians' personal experiences and family legacies of loss. Our own resilience is tested in work with loss; by engaging openheartedly and bringing forth clients' strengths and potential alongside their struggles, this work can be profoundly meaningful for helping professionals as well as for our clients.

CHAPTER 6

Loss Across
the Family Life Cycle

Death of a Spouse, Parent, Child, Sibling

> You will lose someone you can't live without, and your heart
> will be badly broken, and the bad news is that you never
> completely get over the loss . . . But this is also the good
> news. They live forever in your broken heart that doesn't seal
> back up. And you come through. It's like having a broken leg
> that never heals perfectly—that still hurts when the weather
> gets cold, but you learn to dance with the limp.
> —ANNE LAMOTT

A family life-cycle perspective enables clinicians to understand how
the timing of a loss intersects with salient developmental issues and transitions in individual, couple, and family life passage. In this chapter, we'll
address bereavement challenges in couples, in families raising children,
and in adulthood and later life, with the death of a spouse, parent, child,
sibling, and grandparent or grandchild.

THE FAMILY SYSTEM EVOLVING THROUGH TIME

The family, as a relational system, evolves over the life course and across
the generations. Families construct and reweave a complex web of kinship
ties within and across households, linking past, present, and future as they
move forward in life passage. Relationships with parents, siblings, spouses,
children, and other family members grow and change, boundaries shift,
roles are redefined, and new members and losses require adaptation.

As noted in earlier chapters, a death in the family involves multiple losses: the person who died, the meaning of each relationship, missing role functions, and a unique position. Death poses shared adaptational challenges involving both immediate and long-term family reorganization and changes in a family's identity and purpose (Shapiro, 1994).

Individual and family development are intertwined, with each life phase and transition posing new challenges and opportunities. Parental priorities intersect with their children's developmental needs, which differ among siblings. The impact of a death in the family will likely vary for individual members and for a couple or family unit, depending on their concurrent life-phase-related priorities and stresses.

THE TIMING OF LOSS

Past developmental models of normative, progressive life stages have been expanded to recognize the broad diversity in family patterns, relational bonds, and individual life passages (Walsh, 2012). Still, it is helpful to understand salient issues that commonly emerge for those dealing with loss at various life phases and transitions. The timing of a loss in family life may increase the risk for complicated bereavement. As noted in Chapter 5, a family genogram and timeline (McGoldrick et al., 2020) are useful tools to track the sequence and concurrence of losses with other nodal events or stressors and symptoms of distress.

Sudden, Unanticipated Loss

A death that occurs out of the blue is shocking and disorganizing. "It was an ordinary day." "I never imagined." "She was in perfect health." One couple was on a Sunday stroll in their neighborhood when the husband suddenly collapsed and died of a massive heart attack. Most loved ones are totally unprepared: "We meant to discuss our advance directives, our finances and a will, but just didn't get around to it." Many have painful regrets, often carrying them for years: "I would have made an effort to see my dad if I had known there'd never be another chance"; "I wouldn't have had that fight with her the night before if I'd known she wouldn't be coming back"; "Did she know I loved her?"

Untimely Losses

Deaths are harder to bear when they are premature or off time from chronological or social expectations for life trajectories, particularly early spousal loss, early parent loss, or the death of a child. Many families struggle with a sense of injustice when a life—and relationships—are lost too soon, dashing future hopes and dreams.

Concurrence of Losses with Other Major Transitions, Multiple Stressors

The concurrence of loss with other major stressors, posing incompatible demands and cumulative strains, can overload family functioning and interfere with grief (Walsh & McGoldrick, 2004). Complications are more likely when bereavement coincides with other family developmental transitions, particularly with marriage, childbirth, launching of young adults, divorce, or remarriage and stepfamily formation.

With a new marriage or baby at the time of a loss, joy and grief commonly commingle. Yet unaddressed mourning can interfere with investment in the new relationship. Our early clinical studies found that the concurrence of a significant death with the birth of a child posed risks of attachment complications when the grief was unattended, with later difficulties for the offspring in separation and young adult pursuits (Walsh & McGoldrick, 1991). Children fared well in families that supported both the parent's grief and the newborn's needs.

Reactivation of Past Traumatic Loss

Painful memories and emotions from past traumatic losses can be aroused at a current developmental milestone, precipitating a highly distressing crisis (see Chapter 10). Therapists need to explore past losses that may influence expectations, such as catastrophic fears of death or of spousal or child loss at the same age that a past traumatic death occurred in the family, even a generation earlier.

Loss at Different Phases in the Family Life Cycle

The impact of loss can vary with individual and family developmental challenges (Walsh & McGoldrick, 2013). A few salient issues are noted next to suggest the complex interplay of the influences of loss for couples; for children, parents, and siblings in childrearing families; and for those in middle and later life.

COUPLES AND LOSS OF A SPOUSE

Couples today, less bound by family traditions, develop a wide range of intimate committed bonds across racial, cultural, and religious backgrounds and a broad spectrum in gender identity and sexual orientation. Losing the love of one's life can be devastating, as Joan Didion experienced in the sudden death of her husband, her constant companion and support (Didion, 2005). Her grief became all the more unbearable when their daughter later died within the year.

For many, grief with loss after a lengthy, debilitating illness may be complicated by guilt-tinged relief at the end of caregiving burdens. Additionally, negotiating complex extended family relationships at a time of spousal loss can be fraught, as in stepfamilies or where a family of origin has disapproved of a bond, especially for gender-nonconforming couples from more conservative families and faiths.

Early Spousal Loss

Loss of a spouse in young adulthood can be highly disruptive, completely out of sync with life-course expectations and with lives of peers. Hopes and dreams for a shared future or for starting a family are derailed. It can be a shocking and isolating experience without emotional preparation or social support. Socializing with other couples can be awkward and uncomfortable. After initial condolences, peers often distance to avoid confronting their own mortality or possible loss of their partner. Fears of a lonely life ahead lead some—more often men—to repartner rapidly, sometimes within months. For those raising children, suddenly on their own, well-intentioned relatives may encourage a precipitous replacement to provide support and a second parent for children. Yet, plunging into a new intimate relationship to avoid the pain of loss risks carrying unaddressed mourning and attachment issues into the new relationships (as we saw for Maureen and her partner in Chapter 5). In some cases, intense emotions from the earlier loss unexpectedly surface later with relational breakup. In other cases, catastrophic fears of another loss can lead to avoidance or retreat from other intimate partner commitments. Often it is the later crisis that brings them to therapy (see Chapter 10). It's important for therapists to explore reverberations from the past spousal loss.

The term *widowhood* can be problematic, conjuring a lonely life and status set in stone. The label of *widow* should not define the survivor's identity. It's important to challenge outdated and negative stereotypes, for example, that (re)marriage is necessary for one to be fulfilled. The experience of early spousal loss is deeply painful. Yet most widowed persons forge satisfying lives over time, some with new intimate partners and others remaining on their own, valuing job and personal priorities and family, social, and community connections.

Spousal Bereavement in Middle and Later Life

For all couples, loss is inevitable: one partner will most likely die before the other. Yet, spousal loss at midlife, as in earlier loss, is untimely and less commonly experienced by peers who may distance, unready to confront their own mortality or survivorship. Few plan or discuss end-of-life wishes or arrangements for survivors. For childrearing couples, the loss of a partner is complicated by financial and parenting concerns. Typically, as children leave home, most couples reinvest energy in their relationship, with anticipation of shared plans, such as travel and retirement. The death of a partner shatters those dreams. The bereaved spouse may also be reluctant to burden adult children pursuing their dreams or raising children. We encourage women and men to gain perspective on their own lives: to consider how they will manage on their own, develop meaningful pursuits, and build a supportive social network for the years ahead.

> Denise, in her late 40s, came for help after the sudden death of her husband at age 52. They had never imagined the possibility of their death or widowhood. She had relied on his money management throughout their marriage and was overwhelmed by the confusing array of paperwork and financial matters she would need to manage. Through therapeutic coaching sessions, she got in touch with the competencies she had had before marriage, which she said "were like muscles she hadn't exercised in years." This analogy helped her to persist in attempts to regain and build on her skills. Finding she enjoyed the process, she returned to college to forge a new career.

Spousal bereavement in later life can be a highly stressful transition (Carr & Jeffreys, 2010). Adaptation is influenced by the quality of the relationship and by the nature of the death, which most often occurs after prolonged challenges of chronic illness and disability (Rolland, 2018). After a long marriage, most widowed individuals experience profound grief and initial challenges in daily living in the first year. Sleeping alone, having morning coffee in silence, and interrupted daily rhythms are all constant reminders of a shared life lost. Over 1 to 2 years, most surviving spouses adapt well and are quite resilient, becoming more competent and independent, and valuing bonds with family, friends, faith communities, and companion animals.

Clinicians can foster positive adaptation by facilitating grief processes and encouraging supportive connections, while cautioning the bereaved to pace decisions and relocations. Those who have experienced anticipatory loss in caring for a spouse through a long, debilitating illness and disability, especially involving cognitive decline, may be ready to move on more quickly to new relationships and life possibilities. It's important to explore their caregiving experience, appreciate their burdens or sacrifices, and humanize, as common and understandable, their readiness to move forward and any guilt about their relief or surviving and flourishing in life.

Studies of heterosexual marriages find that women, with a longer life expectancy than men and often younger than their male partner, are more likely to be widowed, with many years ahead. Their long-term hardships are compounded by more limited financial resources. Men tend to be less prepared for spousal loss and often have minimized their dependency needs. As one man lamented after his wife, 7 years younger, died, "I always assumed I'd be the first to go. I never expected to be alone—I don't know how to live without her." Men often have greater initial difficulty in coping and are at increased risk of illness, death, and suicide in the first year of bereavement, with the sense of loss, disorientation, and loneliness and the loss of companionship and spousal caregiving (Ennis & Majid, 2021). Older widowed men are less likely to have close male friends or comfort in emotional sharing, and their relational contacts are often more disrupted by retirement and the loss of their wives, who maintained their links to family and social networks. Not surprisingly, remarriage is more common for older American men. Many widowed women prefer not to remarry, especially after heavy spousal caregiving responsibilities and with reluctance to take on that role again. Economic and legal issues, such as bequests for children, lead some repartnered couples to live together without legal status. Many prefer to be committed companions, keeping separate residences and finances, a growing trend termed Living Apart Together (LAT).

The adaptational challenges in spousal loss involve grieving the loss of one's life partner, regaining ongoing functioning, and reinvesting in other relationships and meaningful pursuits. Common tasks include acknowledging the reality of the death and transforming shared daily experiences into memories and deeds. Open expression of grief and loss is important as well as attention to the demands of daily functioning, self-support, household management, and adjustment to being physically and emotionally alone. Other dislocations compound the challenges, particularly when a disabled person has lost their caregiving spouse and must give up their home and community.

In the first year, feelings of loneliness and yearning tend to predominate; yet each situation is unique. I once worked with a woman whose depression lifted after her husband's recent death. She had suffered his controlling and belittling treatment over the years, but being devoutly religious, she couldn't divorce him. She admitted she had often prayed to God to please end her misery, and finally her prayers were answered.

Despite profound initial grief and challenges in daily living, most surviving spouses are quite resilient over time. Most report becoming more competent and independent and take pride in coping well; only a few view the changes entirely negatively. A realignment of intergenerational relationships also occurs as attention turns to the demands of daily functioning and needed support by adult children or other caregivers.

Whenever possible, clinicians and adult children should encourage both partners to plan and discuss end-of-life arrangements, and to anticipate and prepare for widowhood. Many need to acquire new competencies and social supports for independent living. The initial adjustment to being physically alone is in itself difficult. Further dislocation occurs if their home is given up when limited finances, illness, or disabilities preclude independent living. Many are "between a rock and a hard place": reluctant to move in with adult children and burden them, but not wanting to move to a nursing home either. Family consultation can be useful to discuss needs and ways to meet healthcare, economic, and residential challenges.

LOSS IN CHILDREARING FAMILIES

In childrearing families, the death and loss of a significant family member disrupts family life as it affects all surviving members and their bonds.

Death of a Parent

The death of a parent in two-parent families is complicated by the need to realign roles and resources as single-parent households. The surviving parent experiences a double loss: of their life partner and their coparent. Combined job, financial, and childrearing demands can deplete the sole parent's energy and interfere with grief. As children commonly worry about losing their surviving parent, some cover their grief by comforting or supporting a bereaved parent; some may draw attention to distract, such as clowning or misbehaving. Strong support from extended family members and friends is essential to enable the parent to grieve and have respite from demands.

Some children who lose a parent early in life suffer long-term emotional difficulties, with trouble forming intimate attachments and catastrophic fears of separation and abandonment. But most children are not doomed to future difficulties, as longitudinal research makes clear. Children's bereavement and long-term adaptation are influenced not only by the attachment and degree of care lost, but also by the care they receive and

what happens as their lives proceed after the loss. Most fare well in financially secure single-parent homes where there is strong caregiver functioning and extended kin support. Their healing and resilience depend most
on how the family helps them to deal with the death and on the coordination of family life in the aftermath (Greeff & Human, 2004).

With the death of a parent, family structure can break down; leadership, role functioning, and communication may falter. It is crucial for the
family to buffer short-term disruptions for children and other vulnerable
members, reconfigure their home situation, and provide daily structure,
warm nurturance, and continuity in school, peer, and other involvements
(Walsh, 2016c). Parental death can disrupt family units, shifting members
into new and varied relational and household patterns. Adults need to
provide clear information and reassurance that children will be well cared
for and not be abandoned. Efforts should also be made to keep siblings
together, or in regular contact, so that they do not also lose this vital bond.
Reliable contact with a surviving parent is most important when living
apart.

In most cultures, with a parent loss, older children are expected to
take on more responsibilities to support the surviving parent and family
functioning. (Therapists should not assume this is pathological parentifica-
tion, an early family systems concept.) It can build competencies in youth,
as long as expectations are age-appropriate and their own developmental
needs are not neglected. Yet, a child may be overburdened if expected to
replace the lost parent's role, often gendered, such as "man of the house."
An older daughter may be expected to take over childrearing, cooking,
and housework. Therapists can foster both child and family resilience by
facilitating a resource team approach: building cohesion and collaboration
by involving children and other members in contributing to shared efforts.

With the death of a single parent, clinicians can be helpful in assessing
the feasibility and benefits in living with a nonresidential parent, grandparents, or other relatives. Most important, within and across residences,
is the assurance of reliable, caring, and secure contact and for children not
to feel abandoned. Most children do well in kinship care, typically with
grandparents; yet older caregivers' own health, financial challenges, or
conflicting responsibilities should be considered. It can be valuable to convene a family meeting with all involved adult members to assess residential
options and facilitate decisions that will assure children's nurturing care.
Because siblings' bonds are so important in the adaptation of bereaved
children, arrangements should be made to keep them together or, at least,
assure ongoing contact.

Sometimes well-intentioned relatives or friends encourage a surviving parent to rush into a new marriage—and even suggest candidates—to
fill a missing parental role for children. This can complicate their shared

grief experience and children's acceptance of a new stepparent, as in the following case:

> Bill was raising his children, 16-year-old Cal and 14-year-old Rose, on his own after the death of their mother 18 months earlier. He sought therapy for Rose's stormy oppositional behavior with him. In the first session, focused on the current family unit, the problem was initially assessed as a triangle in which the father's strong bond with Cal excluded Rose, who then sought attention through misbehavior. The next few sessions with Bill aimed, unsuccessfully, to strengthen his parenting skills and attachment with Rose.
>
> Unseen beyond the borders of the household and immediate time frame were critical relational complications fueling the crisis. In a family consultation, we learned that within months of the mother's death, Bill had begun a new intimate relationship with Donna, who was now pressuring him to marry. He was ambivalent and dragging his feet. Cal was supportive, wanting his dad to be happy, but Rose repeatedly rebuffed Donna's efforts to win over her affections.
>
> In a family session with Bill and his children, we explored the impact of the mother's death. Rose expressed upset with her father for not helping her or Cal with their grief and began to cry. Cal nodded silently and reached out to take her hand. Their father acknowledged that he had barely grieved himself, saying he had so many obligations to take care of—and it was just too painful. Rose shouted, "Then how could you jump into bed so fast with Donna?! You dishonored Mom!" She also resented Donna for "trying so hard to be our 'replacement' mom." Bill expressed his regrets and vowed to do better. These relational knots needed to be untangled for Bill and his children to grieve their loss before moving forward into a new marriage and stepfamily.

With individual grief and shared adaptational challenges in a family, sending members to separate individual therapists can add complications without close communication. Systemic therapists prefer to combine individual and joint sessions, with the same therapist or a coordinated team approach, to address both personal and relational issues and build mutual support.

> Over the next 10 weeks, the therapist met individually with Bill to focus on his spousal bereavement and challenges as a sole parent and held individual and joint sessions with Rose and Cal to address the loss of their mother. Family sessions with their father then helped them to share their grief, find ways to honor the memory of their mother, and build mutual support in knitting together their single-parent family unit. The father continued to see Donna, clearer with her that he and

his children needed more time to absorb their loss, before making any future commitments.

Bonds with companion animals can be vital supports for children's resilience through family turmoil with loss (Walsh, 2009a, 2009b). In the aftermath of parent loss, further disruptive separations, household instability and confusion, or lack of protection for children heighten their risk of problems.

> Amber's whole life was upended at age 7, when her father died of kidney disease. Her mother, financially strapped and unable to afford their rent, packed up their belongings in their van, and they moved to another town to live with relatives. At Amber's pleading, she let her take her dog. Over the following year, Sparky was Amber's constant, comforting support in grieving her father's loss, in missing her home, friends, school, and neighborhood, and in adapting to a new life. Sparky's doggy antics also gave them shared enjoyment and laughter amid their hardships.

Because social supports often dwindle soon after a loss, links with kin and community throughout the first year are important to contribute to role functions lost, support a bereaved spouse/caregiver, and give attention to children. The potential role of aunts, uncles, and godparents—historically important when early parental death was so common—should be considered. Brief group interventions for parentally bereaved children can have positive effects.

Facilitating Children's Adaptation to Loss in the Family

Children's response to death will depend on their emotional and cognitive development, on the attachment and care they have lost, on the way adults deal with them around the death, and on how they are cared for in the aftermath. Children's reactions are frequently a barometer of family upset, expressing the unspeakable or drawing needed attention to family concerns. If parents are struggling with their own emotional loss, a child may draw fire by misbehavior.

It's important for adults to recognize both the curiosity and limitations in a child's ability to understand what is happening and not to be alarmed by seemingly unemotional or "inappropriate" responses. Children need help in comprehending the loss experience at their developmental level. They seek understanding by observing the reactions of adult relatives. Therapists can encourage families to keep communication open to many conversations over time to facilitate understanding and address other concerns as they mature. When a mother dies of breast cancer, an

8-year-old daughter may be intensely grieving her loss; with her development at puberty, anxiety may arise that she, too, might die from breast cancer.

Very young children don't understand that death is final. Most believe it is reversible or temporary, and they may ask repeatedly where the deceased has gone and when they're coming back. Curious about the world, they see death on television and social media, arousing questions about death that may make adults uncomfortable. Magical thinking is common, and they see movie, cartoon, or internet characters die and come back. They may not show outward signs of grieving, or they may only react intermittently because they expect a loved one's return.

Some children become angry at the deceased for leaving or at a surviving parent or sibling. Some worry that their anger or naughty behavior caused the death. Some show clinging behavior, afraid someone else will disappear. Parents may need help in understanding variable responses and easing unrealistic expectations for them to comprehend death and loss. We can encourage them to be attentive to nonverbal and symbolic forms of expression.

School-age children vary widely in response. With developing cognitive abilities, most are better able to understand that death is final and that it will happen to everyone someday. But only imagining it vaguely, or in the far-off future, they may be shocked by an actual death and may even act as if it did not occur. Some show little reaction but become overly helpful in attending to others' grief. Some, not differentiating clearly between thoughts and actions, may believe that their anger or rivalry caused a death. Some develop somatic symptoms or heightened anxiety with a fear of death. Those who hide sad feelings to act mature and not seem childish may instead express anger or irritability.

To support children after a death, open communication is vital. While it is natural to want to protect a child, honesty and transparency build trusting bonds and coping ability. Child guidance experts (e.g., *www.unicel.org*) generally recommend encouraging the following guidelines for families:

• Tell the truth, without delay, and validate children's feelings and concerns. Share sad news and information sensitively, in a safe, quiet place, and help them to gain comprehension. Try to respond simply, avoid euphemisms, and clarify ambiguities: A parent "passed away" or "left us" doesn't mean they went on a trip and may (or may not) be coming back. Telling what happened in traumatic deaths, including homicide or suicide, is important, in age-appropriate ways. It's better to acknowledge any ambiguity in the situation, rather than saying nothing until certain, and to assure children that parents will share more information as it becomes clearer. If a child is anxious about death and threatened loss or asks, "when are you (or am I) going to die?" families can assure them that they will do all they can to take good care of themselves and each other.

• Help children to feel included in the family mourning process. Most do better when they are involved in funeral or memorial events rather than being left on the sidelines. Involve them later in planning and participation to honor the deceased on anniversaries, holidays, and birthdays.

• Normalize varied experiences in children's grief processes over time: they may be affected physically (sickness, headaches, sleep difficulties); emotionally (sad, mad, empty, scared); cognitively (concentration, focus); behaviorally (withdrawal, sensitivity, misbehavior); or spiritually (prayer, questioning or talking to God, asking what happens after death).

• Children need time to absorb the news. They may appear not to hear or understand and ask the same questions repeatedly. Parents need to be patient and open to many conversations, helping them understand that grief takes time and that painful feelings, such as sadness, anger, or fears, may come out in small spurts or arise later unexpectedly. Naming and talking about their feelings is helpful. Let them see your sadness and reassure them that there is nothing wrong with sharing feelings with others. Reassure them that it's also OK to experience joyful times amid sorrows, to want time alone and with friends. Encourage peer and social contacts.

• Children process their grief through imagination, play, and creative activity. Children's books and videos about death and loss (including classics such as *Charlotte's Web* and *Mister Rogers' Neighborhood* PBS episode "Death of a Goldfish" for young children) can be helpful resources to discuss together. Parents can encourage expression through different outlets, such as journaling. Art expression and play therapy techniques, such as sand play, are valuable in advancing children's emotional processing, meaning making, and relational connection (Gil, 2014). Family play therapy harnesses the family's inherent abilities to access and utilize their strengths for healing and growth from painful loss experiences

For adolescents, the developmental impetus toward autonomy can interfere with their acknowledgment of the significance of a parental loss. Heated conflicts over authority or wishes to be rid of parental control may spark guilt when a parent dies, complicating bereavement, with mixed feelings and minimization of the loss.

Jesse, age 38, came for therapy around his repeated job losses due to his heated conflicts with his bosses. Asked about his family relationships, he shared that in adolescence, he had defied his father's authority and fought bitterly with his father over control issues; when his father died in an industrial accident, he had barely grieved and left home soon after, putting it all behind him.

Adolescents may retreat from family interaction following a death, isolating themselves in their rooms, often immersing themselves in video games and social media. They may rebuff parents' attempts to engage them, and they may not talk to anyone about the experience. Fostering trusting bonds, reliable structure, and open communication can enable them to share concerns. Many teens want to discuss questions about death and the meaning of life, suggesting the importance of conversations that help them clarify their beliefs (Walsh, 2009c). Longitudinal studies find that strong sibling bonds contribute to better life trajectories after experiences of adverse events. Gender and age difference matter less than mutual respect, cooperation, and encouragement in managing difficulties.

Teenagers commonly turn to friends for support. Those lacking strong family resources are more vulnerable to negative peer influences and may try to escape the pain of loss through high-risk behavior. In turn, their defiance of parental concerns and controls further stresses the bereaved family. As school or juvenile authorities tend to focus on problem behavior, it's crucial to explore the influence of recent losses and assist youths and their families in addressing them.

Death of a Child

The death of a child is the most tragic of all untimely losses, reversing the natural order of life passage and shattering parents' (and elders') future hopes and dreams. Their sense of injustice can arouse profound questioning of the meaning of life. Some turn away from their faith in God (see Chapter 3). The anguish of loved ones can interfere with their life pursuits and cast a shadow over joys for years to come. As one mother lamented, "You cannot fast forward through grief to get to the other side; there is no other side when it's your child. You carry the love and the loss with you for the rest of your life."

In working with parental grief, it's important to assess and encourage supportive relational connections, which can be vital in adaptation (Bartel, 2020). Many parents find that investing energy in surviving children can facilitate positive adaptation. The common impetus to have another child can bring solace, and yet it does not replace the one who died. As one mother said, "I love my daughter, yet the absence of my son will always be there." Therapy can be helpful if intense and debilitating grief persists.

Parents commonly face painful social situations when asked, "How many children do you have?" Do they mention the child they lost? One mother worried about her surviving child's dilemma: "My daughter is an only child, yet she isn't. How will she answer the question through life: 'Do you have brothers and sisters?' How will she draw the picture of her family?" Whom do you tell? How much do you tell? Therapists can help families consider ways they might deal with such questions, depending on the situation and how much they prefer to share.

Of all losses, it is hardest not to idealize a child who has died. Grief may intensify at nodal points, such as the graduation of the child's peers. A number of studies have documented the high distress of bereaved parents in depression, anxiety, somatic symptoms, self-esteem, and sense of control in life. Particularly difficult can be the death of the firstborn, an only child, the only son or daughter, a gifted child, or one with special needs. Because small children are so utterly dependent on parents for their safety and survival, parental blame and guilt can be especially strong in accidental deaths or an unclear cause, such as SIDS (sudden infant death syndrome). Blame is particularly likely to fall on mothers, who are expected to carry the primary responsibility for children's well-being.

The death of an adolescent is heartbreaking for families, having nurtured their youth almost to adulthood. Parents commonly carry intense sadness, anger, and despair about the loss of a young life of promise. With life-threatening illnesses, such as diabetes or cancer, adolescents' defiance of treatment regimens can spark battles with parents and heighten their lethal risks (Rolland, 2018). With their death, family grief can be fraught with anger at the youth and parental conflict with guilt and mutual recriminations.

The most common adolescent deaths are from accidents, suicide, and homicide, which are all traumatic losses for the family (see Chapter 9). They are often complicated by impulsive, risk-taking behavior and are encouraged by peers. Possible family influences, such as violence, sexual abuse, or past traumatic deaths should be explored (see Chapter 10). The high risk of suicide by gender-nonconforming teens and others who face peer bullying is significantly lower for those with family acceptance (Haas et al., 2010). In neighborhoods plagued by violence and drugs, youth-on-youth homicides take a tragic toll, and bereaved families grapple with intense anger, frustration, and despair (see Chapter 11).

Impact of Child Loss in Couple Relationships

The marital relationship is particularly vulnerable to breakdown with a child's death (Stroebe, Schut, & Finkenauer, 2013). However, the data are mixed: most couples weather the tragedy, and many report strengthened bonds through their mutual support through the ordeal. Bereavement is eased when both parents have participated in taking care of a sick child prior to death and when they share a philosophy of life or strong faith beliefs that offer meaning and comfort. Family therapy can be valuable in strengthening their relationship through a terminal illness and in the aftermath, bolstering mutual support, respect for different coping responses, and good communication and collaboration (Kissane et al., 2016). Bereavement groups can provide a supportive network for dealing with the painful experience of child loss (Sandler, Wolchik, Ayers, Tein, & Luecken, 2013). It's important to involve fathers, as groups are commonly attended by mothers, with few fathers participating.

Impact of Child Death for Siblings

The needs of siblings may be neglected when a child dies, especially after a protracted illness and caregiving demands. They often suffer quietly on the sidelines, not wanting to further burden parents. With the death of a sibling, survivor guilt is common: Why them and not me? How can I be happy when they died?

One child survived a car crash with barely a scratch when their sibling, sitting next to them, did not. In some cases, normal sibling rivalry contributes to survival guilt, blocking developmental strivings well into adulthood. One might believe that they somehow caused a death, as through rough play, jealousy, or wishes to be rid of a rival for parental attention. Some carry the fear that they will also die in the same way, becoming overly anxious about a headache or virus. After a death in high-risk circumstances, some siblings become avoidant of similar situations; others may seek them out to tempt or defy fate. Parents' own anxieties and overprotection of siblings can intensify the situation (see Chapter 10). One mother couldn't let her daughter out of her sight whenever they went out, years after an older daughter had been hit and killed in traffic. Therapists can help families discuss such concerns and reasonable precautions.

In some cases, bereaved parents withdraw from surviving children to avoid being vulnerable to loss again. In some cases a sibling may assume a replacement role for the family to avoid the pain of loss. However, if the child's own needs and unique attributes are not affirmed, later attempts at separation and individuation may impair the young person's development and precipitate delayed grief responses in parents (McGoldrick & Walsh, 1983).

Small children commonly use magical thinking and invent imaginary friends or siblings to help them cope with traumatic loss experiences, as in the following situation of sibling loss. Clinicians can normalize and encourage parental understanding and support of such expression.

> One father related the experience of his 3-year-old daughter, Ella, as her baby sister went through months of treatment for a brain tumor and then died. Supported by her parents, Ella visited her sister in the hospital, pleased to make her smile. One day, she began talking about an imaginary brother, named Mingus. She would tell her parents stories about how he had a tumor and how she would give him shots and treatments to get better. After her baby sister died, she informed her parents that Mingus had moved out—but he was living around the corner. Occasionally, she would report visits and conversations with Mingus, and how she was glad he wasn't in pain anymore.
>
> Her father, a writer from Bosnia, had written accounts of the ethnic cleansing atrocities experienced by his community. Now, in suffering their family tragedy, he appreciated her ability to construct imaginary stories as a way to process mentally and emotionally all that was happening that was beyond her comprehension and control. As he dealt with his own grief over the following months, he decided to write about the experience they had all come through, stressing that he was doing this not for himself but to bear witness to their experience and honor the baby's short life (Hemon, 2014).

Grandparent Loss

The death of a grandparent is commonly children's first experience in learning how to deal with a significant loss. Grandparents and grandchildren often enjoy a special bond, not complicated by the responsibilities and conflicts in parent–child relationships. Adolescents are often less ambivalent and more openly expressive of sadness in missing a grandparent. When the grandparent has served a central role in the family and in childrearing, commonly in African American, Native American, and immigrant families and in kinship care placements, the loss is more profound in both the youth's emotional bond and family functioning (Hayslip & Kaminski, 2005). However, a conflictual parent–grandparent relationship, often over authority or child loyalties, can complicate grief.

LOSS IN ADULTHOOD AND LATER LIFE

The impact of parental loss in adulthood is often underestimated. As children leave home in emerging adulthood, the family experiences a major transition as intergenerational and spousal relationships are realigned and the household is reorganized. Parents at midlife confront losses on both sides, with children leaving and aging parents declining in health and dying. For generations in middle and later life, the growing frequency of deaths of loved ones and peers heightens awareness of the inevitability of loss and their own mortality.

Impact of Parental Loss for Young Adults

For young adults, a parent's death and related family needs and obligations can impact educational aims or newly initiated career or relationship pursuits. Adult life plans may be sidelined by expectations to provide financial or emotional support, to become the head of the family or carry on a family business, or to provide care for a surviving parent. Some need to move back home, take in a widowed parent, or arrange their long-term care.

Yet, with Western societal expectations for emerging adults to emancipate, the meaning and significance of the bond for them may be unrecognized, and their own loss and grief may be minimized by the young person, their families, friends, and even therapists (see Chapter 12). Others who are not yet secure on their own may be highly anxious about making their way without parental support. Caution is needed for those who seek emotional security through replacement in a new intimate bond.

Impact of Parental Loss in Couple Relationships

The death of a parent in one's family of origin can stoke tensions or embed complicated mourning issues in a couple's bond. A partner's sense of responsibility to their parents may generate conflicts in loyalty and attention. In cross-cultural marriages, a Euro-American spouse expecting the marriage to come first may not understand that their partner, from a Latinx culture, for example, may be expected to place intergenerational bonds and obligations over spousal investment (Falicov, 2014). Fostering mutual understanding and support can facilitate mourning and strengthen relational resilience.

Extensive caregiving or support to the dying or surviving parent can strain the couple's bond. The combined stress and grief often disrupt sexual desire, affecting intimacy. Attachment injuries can occur if the bereaved person feels unsupported or if their partner feels neglected over an extended period of time (Johnson, 2019).

> Paula and Kevin came to couple therapy increasingly estranged. Paula complained that Kevin was just not there for her when she really needed him. The therapist asked if there was a particular time that she needed him badly and felt he wasn't responsive. Paula teared up, recalling her father's sudden death, 2 years earlier. He was the strong one in the family, whom everyone depended on. Her mother fell apart, so Paula, an only child, had to take care of all funeral and financial matters and then tend to her mother's needs, making all arrangements for her to move out of the family home to assisted living. With the cumulative stresses over many months, Paula was physically exhausted and emotionally depleted. She sought individual therapy, which helped to process her grief, but the contrast of her therapist's compassionate understanding with Kevin's remoteness increased her anger and withdrawal from him. She sobbed, "Kevin, I needed *you* to take care of me, even just to hold me through it all. But you were always too busy. I felt so alone in the world."
>
> Kevin moved close to her and put his arms around her, holding her as she sobbed. He apologized, and said, "I didn't realize how much you needed me—you're so competent, like your father, and always know how to take charge of tough situations. You seemed to be managing it all. I felt I was just in the way . . . and I didn't know what to do—except not to burden you with my own needs. So, I just stuffed them and backed off to give you space to do everything you had to do. I don't mean to excuse it; I wasn't there for you and I'm so sorry."
>
> In the following sessions, Kevin also revealed his sense of inadequacy in their marriage. Knowing how much Paula and her mother admired the father's financial success, he believed they were both disappointed in him, that he didn't live up to their expectations. The glowing accolades for the father at his funeral brought his insecurity to the fore. His discomfort with his mother-in-law, who tended to find fault with him, contributed to his staying uninvolved with Paula's arrangements for her mother's move.
>
> Paula responded that she loved him in ways in which he was *unlike* her father, especially in his devotion to their children, since her father was rarely there for her growing up. In fact, it was at her father's death, when she desperately needed Kevin's support, that his withdrawal reminded her of her father's unavailability. She acknowledged that maybe she hadn't let him know her needs, since she grew up handling things on her

own so she wouldn't need help that wouldn't be there for her. Her long-submerged anger at her father exacerbated her disappointment in Kevin. Couple therapy was helpful in strengthening their bond, with more open communication, mutual understanding, and support.

Parent Loss in Middle and Later Life

With the death of their parents, adults at midlife typically confront their own mortality and think more about the time that remains ahead of them. The death of the last surviving member of the oldest generation is a family milestone, with the next generation becoming the family elders. It also brings awareness that they are the next expected to die. Having children and grandchildren commonly eases the acceptance of mortality; there may be pressure on the younger generation to start a family. Encouraging other forms of generativity and satisfaction can be meaningful for many.

Most adults in their middle years expect to assume increased responsibilities for aging parents and to accept their deaths as a natural, inevitable occurrence in the life cycle. Yet the demands can be heavy: Most elderly persons die after a long, progressively worsening illness and disability (see Chapter 4). An adult child may be overstressed by pulls in two directions: juggling job and childrearing demands with responsibilities for the dying and surviving parent.

With population trends worldwide—adult children often living at a distance; most women, traditionally the primary caregivers, in the workforce; and a declining birthrate—fewer children and grandchildren are available to attend to dying and widowed elders. With increasing life expectancy, adult children over age 65, with their own declining health and resources, are called upon to care for frail and widowed parents in their 90s. The demand for affordable, quality, long-term and continuing care is critical.

Death of an Adult Child

The death of an adult child before family elders, upending family life-cycle expectations, is especially hard to bear. As a Chinese proverb expresses, "White hair should never follow black [to the grave]." Parents and grandparents commonly experience a sense of injustice in the ending of a life they have nurtured to adulthood. For families that have lovingly raised a child with serious medical, developmental, or mental health conditions, their death can be a particularly wrenching experience.

Loss and Adult Sibling Relationships

Challenges in adult sibling relationships are common with the death or threatened loss of their parent. While gender norms are changing, daughters are more likely stressed by cultural expectations to be primary parental caregivers, while sons tend to shoulder more of the financial responsibilities but less often the day-to-day demands. Sibling sessions can be helpful in addressing burdens or resentments in disparities. For an only child, the overload can interfere with their grieving process. A family systems approach broadens the individual caregiver model to involve family members and others as a collaborative *caregiving team*, each contributing according to abilities, proximity, and resources (Walsh, 2016c). A few joint sessions, with those at a distance participating remotely, can help to air concerns or grievances, begin to share grief, and build mutual support and teamwork. Siblings typically report that their bonds grew closer as they pulled together to meet end-of-life demands and manage affairs and caregiving in the aftermath.

In some cases, longstanding sibling rivalries erupt in conflict after the death of a parent.

> Maggie, age 72, suffered a deep depression after her 95-year-old father died. She had always tried to please him, yet on his deathbed he had asked only for her sister, whom he had always favored. Most painful for Maggie was that, with his death, she would have no future chance to win his affection.

Disputes over wills and keepsakes can fuel resentments and estrangement for years to come. In one family, intense conflict erupted after the funeral between two sisters; although they lived next door to each other, they refused to have any further contact or allow their children to play together. A year later, they came to therapy to reconcile, after the school reported that their sons were repeatedly fighting on the playground. Where a family business is involved, competitive struggles or cutoffs can ensue over succession decisions, with long-lasting grievances. Yet, in many families, siblings' relationships may improve after parental death. Two brothers who had competed since childhood for their father's meager approval found their relationship freed from old rivalries after his death.

The death of a sibling—for most, one's longest relationship through life—can bring surprisingly intense and complicated grief. It's important to understand the meaning and significance of their bond and the relevance of family dynamics. Parents may expect a sibling to carry the torch for the one who died. However, the surviving sibling may be blocked from realizing their own potential by survivor guilt and conflicting family injunctions to replace, but not surpass, the lost child. It may be years later that they come for therapy, struggling with their untenable situation (see Chapter 10).

Family Challenges and Resilience in Later-Life Losses

Later life is a season of cumulative losses of loved ones, friends, and peers. Some older people withdraw and avoid funerals, so as not to face yet another painful loss and their own approaching death. The family as a system, along with its elder members, confronts major adaptational challenges. Changes with illness, death, and widowhood alter complex relationship patterns, often requiring family support, adjustment to loss, reorientation, and reorganization. Such challenges also present opportunities for relational transformation and growth.

Medical advances and neuroscience findings of neuroplasticity support many possibilities for well-being and resilience into later years. It's important to challenge ageist stereotypes of deterioration and decay. Even when parents become quite frail, losing mental or physical capacities, they should not be labeled as "childlike." With many decades more of life experience, they remain parents to their children in the generational hierarchy. The importance of dignity, respect, and involvement as elders approach life's end is paramount.

Notable with aging and the approach of death and loss is the common search for life's transcendent meaning, as spiritual and existential matters come to the fore (see Chapter 3). Efforts by older adults and their families to integrate the varied experiences of a lifetime into a coherent sense of self, family identity, and a meaningful life can foster intergenerational integrity and adaptation (King & Wynne, 2004). A priority for resilience is to draw out sources of meaning and satisfaction and to integrate the varied experiences of a lifetime into a coherent sense of self, relational integrity, and life's worth. Intergenerational continuities are fostered in passing on positive legacies.

A conjoint family life review (see Chapter 4) can assist family members in sharing reminiscences and gaining understanding of family members' lives and relationships. Members can incorporate multiple perspectives and the subjective experiences of their life passage, enlarging the family story and strengthening bonds. Elders approaching life's end are often more forthright about earlier issues, offering the opportunity to heal old wounds.

Bereavement with Varied Family Structures and Life Course

Today, with the multiplicity of family forms, cultures, and varied life trajectories, a more fluid view of family life is required. Over the life course, some people have two or more marriages and raise children at different developmental phases. Many have periods of single living and cohabitation with intimate partners. Children and parents are likely to transition in and out of household and kinship arrangements over time. Families need to buffer transitions entailing multiple losses and to reconfigure their lives in flexible and complex arrangements.

Therapists need to hold an expanded view of family, considering significant bonds and bereavement processes across the complex network of attachments and losses, in and across households and over time. For instance, in divorced families, the death of the custodial parent may generate conflicts between grandparents and the noncustodial parent over the future rearing of children. Grief over the death of a former spouse or an uninvolved, noncustodial parent may be unexpectedly strong (see Chapter 7) and may be complicated by residual feelings from the divorce or children's sense of abandonment. Parental death in gender-variant families can be complicated by family or religious disapproval and by societal laws that deny death benefits to nonbiological coparents and continuing relationships with children they have raised.

With remarriage, children at different developmental stages, and even in different generations, will have varied bonds and responses to loss. Loyalty conflicts may be strong. Biological and stepchildren may clash over a deceased parent's will or burial decisions: which spouse and family are favored? In one happily remarried couple, both of whom were widowed after a lengthy marriage with children, the partners faced a common dilemma: where to be buried. Each had previously vowed to be buried with their first spouse. With the ingenuity that fosters resilience amid the complexities of relational life, they both decided to be cremated at death, with half their ashes buried with their first spouse and the other half commingled together.

A TIME FOR LOSS; A TIME FOR HEALING

Death and loss pose painful and far-reaching adaptational challenges in families over their life course and across the generations. A developmental systemic framework attends to the reverberations of a death—the circumstances and the matrix of meanings it holds—for all family members, their relationships, and the family as a functional unit, interacting with individual and family life passages.

A systemic practice approach to loss is guided by an appraisal of adaptational challenges, variables that heighten vulnerability and risk, and family processes that foster recovery and resilience. Because clinical attention has tended to focus on dysfunctional patterns, it is important to identify and build family strengths and resources. Interventions may flexibly use or combine individual, couple, and family sessions, as well as multifamily groups, to support positive adaptation. Our work with loss involves supporting bereavement processes as clients reach for ways to make meaning of the loss, put it in perspective, and weave the experience of both loss and renewal into the fabric of individual and relational life passages. The multiple meanings of each death are transformed throughout life and across generations as they are integrated into personal and shared identity and with other life experiences.

The chapters in Part III address the more complex challenges for the bereaved in a range of situations of complicated and traumatic loss (see Table 6.1). Principles and guidelines are offered for therapeutic practice to foster healing and resilience.

TABLE 6.1. Situations of Complex and Traumatic Death and Loss

The meaning and impact of deaths are complicated by variables in the loss situation that require careful assessment and attention.

- *Untimely death.* Deaths that are premature or off time from chronological or social expectations, especially the death of a child, seem unjust and rob future hopes and dreams.
- *Sudden death.* A sense of normalcy and predictability is shattered. Shock, disorganization, and intense emotions are common, with added confusion over unplanned last wishes or financial matters; many suffer painful regrets, unable to say their good-byes or repair hurts, often seeking help years later.
- *Prolonged suffering.* With intense physical or emotional suffering before death, the agony for family members can be great, coupled with guilt, anger, or remorse.
- *Ambiguous loss.* Not knowing if a missing loved one is alive or dead can immobilize families and tear them apart, hoping for the best while fearing the worst. When a loved one suffers progressive dementia, the erosion of personhood and relationships is heartbreaking.
- *Unacknowledged and stigmatized losses.* In disenfranchised grief, the significance of a loss is minimized or hidden, or the cause of death is stigmatized, invalidating grief and denying social support. Isolation, secrecy, blocked communication, and estrangement further complicate adaptation.
- *Violent and traumatic death circumstances.* A violent death, especially in a tragic accident, murder, substance overdose, or suicide, is devastating for loved ones. Intense preoccupation with causal accusations, guilt, or negligence can rupture bonds. A senseless tragedy is especially hard to bear.
- *Past traumatic experiences.* Past trauma and losses can be aroused in later difficulties in life pursuits or relational conflict, often at significant anniversaries, in other losses, in major life transitions, and across generations.
- *Pileup of effects.* Families can be overwhelmed by the emotional, relational, and functional impact of multiple stressors, prolonged or recurrent trauma, other losses (homes, jobs, communities), and disruptive transitions (e.g., separations, migration).

PART III

Complex and Traumatic Loss Situations

CHAPTER 7

Ambiguous, Unacknowledged, and Stigmatized Losses

Life is not the way it is supposed to be. It is the way it is.
The way you cope with it is what makes the difference.
—VIRGINIA SATIR

The tragic nature or circumstances of a loss, with the lack of support by others, can complicate bereavement, intensifying suffering, affecting other relationships, and constraining adaptation. When the experience of loss is ambiguous or when it is unacknowledged, minimized, or stigmatized, the bereaved commonly feel isolated or even not entitled to grieve.

AMBIGUOUS LOSSES

Ambiguous losses are experiences of significant loss that are not as concrete, clear, or identifiable as losses with death. Ambiguity surrounding loss has been found to block individual and family mourning processes and to generate anxiety and depression (Boss, 1999).

When a Loved One Is Missing

One type of ambiguous loss involves uncertainty about whether a loved one is alive or dead. The lack of clarity is agonizing, as in cases of disappearance, child kidnapping, or political abduction; or of those missing in collective loss situations, such as a disaster, war, or conflict zones (see Chapter 11). In the 2022 Russian invasion of Ukraine, men were taken away from their homes at gunpoint and did not return. Families, holding onto hope that their loved one was still alive, were in anguish imagining their captivity and torture: were they murdered, or might they someday escape? Bodies were found in the streets, in basements, and in mass graves, but many could not be identified. In such agonizing situations, families commonly become consumed by desperate attempts to get critical information to confirm the fate of their loved one. Serious relational conflict can arise over time as some family members press to move on with life despite lingering ambiguity, while others refuse to give up hope of survival, against all odds.

The recovery and identification of a body or remains are crucial for survivors' ability to begin mourning, with religious rites and (re)burial in family plots important to them (Boss, 2017). Identifying remains through a DNA match is vital; even a birthmark or tattoo makes the death "real." Retrieved objects, a ring or nametag, become painful yet valued keepsakes. After a disaster, families struggle in imagining the circumstances of a disappearance, torture, and death, their minds uneasy without clear evidence. In many cases, the full situation may never be completely verified. Healing is fostered by active pursuits of accountability and justice, supported by neighbors and other witnesses who come forward to testify and can now document atrocities with cellphone photos and videos. Therapists can be helpful to families throughout this process, encouraging their fact-finding efforts and their understanding of different members' perspectives when realistic hopes fade. Periodic contact can be supportive in weathering persistent uncertainty as they navigate their path forward.

Losses with Alzheimer's Disease and Other Dementias

The ambiguous loss of a loved one with progressive neurocognitive impairment is heartbreaking, as they increasingly lose psychological functioning and relational connection while remaining physically present (Boss, 1999). Alzheimer's disease and other dementias affect 1 in 10 people over age 65 and nearly half of persons over age 85. Alzheimer's disease has been called "the long good-bye" because of the gradual deterioration of memory, functioning, identity, family roles, and relationships. The irreversible course of this devastating condition can last from a few years to over two decades, with increasing caregiving, psychosocial, and financial strains on the family. In the early stages of the disease, a diagnosis is often unclear. Family members may become frustrated when the individual repeatedly asks the same questions, forgets earlier answers, or prepares a meal and forgets to serve it. Because of their impaired judgment, some make disastrous financial decisions. Over time, mental, physical, and relational capacities are gradually eroded in confusion, disorientation, and loss of control over bodily functions. In "sundowning," they may wander off, get lost, and forget who they are and where they live. Such multistress challenges further complicate grief for caregivers.

It is especially heart wrenching for close family members when they are no longer recognized or are confused with others, even those of another generation or long deceased. Gentle humor can ease some situations. My colleague, Ezra, shared an incident that occurred at his weekly dinner with his parents. As his mother cleared the table and went into the kitchen, his father leaned over to him and said, "Did you see that woman there? If I wasn't a married man, I could really go for her!" Ezra replied, "Dad, you are the luckiest man on earth because you ARE married to her—she's your wife!" They laughed together and his mother enjoyed the compliment.

With limited medical interventions for disease progression, treatment primarily addresses symptom management and custodial care. Most families try to keep their loved one at home as long as possible. Paid caregivers, extended family, and social support networks are crucial in coping with stressful situations, providing respite in dealing with crises. Adult daycare programs offer a therapeutic milieu, with pleasurable contacts and activities, as they relieve family strains. Family psychoeducation provides useful information and management guidelines to reduce stresses and address both functional and relational losses (Rolland, 2018). A few guidelines for relating and communicating can help families reduce frustration, conflict, and alienation, and, just as important, support the dignity and well-being of the person with dementia:

- Gain understanding and compassion for the neurological influence in confusion, memory lapses, and mistakes.
- Make requests respectfully and encourage efforts, without demanding or condescending.
- Avoid accusations, lecturing, blaming, or shaming corrections.
- When confusion sparks anxiety or agitation, calmly reassure or divert attention.

Temporal disorientation, blurring past and present events, is common in later stages of dementia.

Joel, visiting his father, was startled when he related, with great delight, that he had just had lunch with his wife (who had died many years earlier). Rather than correcting him, Joel smiled, appreciating his father's account of the wonderful meal they enjoyed and how beautiful she looked. He died peacefully in his sleep a few weeks later. Joel wondered:

was it his father's past reminiscence or his future hopes of reunion that surfaced in his mind? Either way, his dreamlike account brought joy in the moment.

To foster resilience and enhanced connection, it's important to practice the "art of the possible." Family members can be encouraged to share pleasurable "here and now" moments of relating. It might be through enjoying a tasty snack, finding humor, connecting with nature, appreciating music, and sharing reminiscences with photos and stories that are evoked. It's important to include the person in gatherings while respecting limitations. One grandfather with dementia could no longer follow family conversations but found contentment petting the family dog, snuggled close on the sofa. He took great delight in sneaking sausages under the dinner table to his attentive companion.

In some cases of advanced dementia, the present becomes excruciatingly painful for loved ones, as in the following situation:

Marcia sought therapy in deep depression. Two years earlier she had given up her valued professional career to care for her husband, Charles, as his dementia worsened. When he could no longer be cared for at home, Marcia helped him settle comfortably in a memory care facility and visited him daily. One day she arrived to find that Charles had become romantically involved with another resident, whom he introduced to her as his new love, unaware that Marcia was his wife.

The therapy was helpful in unpacking the many facets of Marcia's grief, including her anger at the loss of her career to care tirelessly for a husband who no longer knew her and now loved another woman. It was helpful to contextualize his extremely hurtful behavior as impacted by his neurological condition. We explored her unfolding experience as a caregiving spouse of a loved one with dementia who gradually slipped away.

Over the following weeks, I encouraged Marcia to bring in old photographs, expanding the therapeutic conversation to explore their life together from their early love and shared hopes and dreams to satisfactions and disappointments over the course of their marriage. This helped her to integrate the painful and challenging recent experiences wrought by Charles's disease as a chapter in the larger story of their marriage in her book of life. I encouraged Marcia to feel entitled to grieve her recent losses and yet to keep precious memories of their love and her husband's abiding loyalty over the years. At our last session, she said that while visits (less frequent) would still be hard, she found comfort in knowing he was happy and in holding onto their memories for both of them.

When a spouse with advanced dementia lives for many years, a caregiving spouse may be wracked with guilt, torn between a desire for intimate companionship with a new partner and an obligation to uphold marital vows—"till death do us part." These are complex dilemmas, involving relational ethics. While some want a therapist to advise them what to do, that is not our role. We can attend to their complicated grief and support their efforts to sort out issues of loyalty, obligation, compassionate caregiving, and self-care. Coaching them for conversations with their adult children can also be important. We can help them gain peace of mind as they chart their way forward. One husband, supported in his own personal decision-making process, knit together a "both/and" plan to honor spousal bonds, continuing to provide sensitive caretaking while also moving forward with a new partner. Yet, each situation is unique.

> Ramon, in his mid-50s, sought help with his painful dilemma. Three years earlier, his husband Richard, the love of his life, had suffered a debilitating brain aneurysm with complications that left him with no recent memory, declining cognitive functioning, and no chance of recovery. Each weekend he drove a long distance to visit Richard at a care facility, but the sadness for both in saying good-bye each time was unbearable and his partner didn't understand why he was not going home. Ramon had become isolated and realized he needed to forge a new personal life and start seeing other people. He said his ideal solution would be to find someone available for "a midweek intimate relationship" so that he could continue to spend weekends with Richard. The therapist, a bit dubious, said it was worth exploring. Indeed, that arrangement did not work out. As the therapy addressed his complicated grief and love for Richard, his desire to remain totally committed became clear. He decided to move closer to the care facility for more frequent visits and to find new avenues for satisfaction in his life.

One should be cautious not to assume that persons with neurocognitive impairment have little comprehension of a significant death. When ways are found to include vulnerable family members in mourning rites, they and their loved ones can benefit, as illustrated in the following situation:

> Abe, age 72, was confined to a nursing home after suffering severe brain damage when hit by a car 5 years earlier. His wife and daughters had to adjust over time to the loss of the husband and father as they had known and loved him. They managed gradually to cope with his profound personality changes, sporadic violent outbursts, and, most painful for them, his recent lapses in recognizing them on visits.

Anticipating his further decline and death, the daughters were unprepared when their mother had a heart attack and died. They wanted their father to be present for her memorial service, but his care facility staff was unwilling to release him, fearing his disruptive behavior (and a possible lawsuit). They insisted that he would not understand that his wife had died and would only become confused and agitated. Determined to include him, the sisters arranged to move the service from the funeral home to the courtyard of his nursing home. They sat on both sides of his wheelchair, their arms around him. Although he initially showed no sign of comprehension, as each sister rose and spoke movingly of their mother's life and death, tears rolled down his cheeks. At the end of the service, he joined in the singing of "Amazing Grace."

UNACKNOWLEDGED AND STIGMATIZED LOSSES: DISENFRANCHISED GRIEF

The term *disenfranchised grief* (Doka, 2002) refers to the experience of losses that may not be openly shared, socially sanctioned, or publicly mourned when unacknowledged, minimized, or stigmatized. Cultural standards strongly influence the experience of bereavement, as in social norms for whom and in what circumstances it is appropriate to grieve (see Chapter 3). Mourning rituals, relational supports, and resources typically offered in socially sanctioned losses may not be available. In turn, the bereaved may be hesitant to express their grief openly or to ask for support. The lack of recognition and validation can contribute to a longer, more intense, and isolated grieving process. In other cases, blocked emotions may go unaddressed, emerging in somatic symptoms, substance use problems, or relational conflict.

Grief may be unacknowledged or stigmatized in varied situations (Werner & Moro, 2004).

1. The loss itself may not be recognized, or it may be minimized, as in a pregnancy–related loss.
2. The significance of the relationship may be underestimated, as in the death of a close friend, classmate, mentor, coworker; a former spouse, or a cherished pet. (For discussion of losing a companion animal, see Chapter 8.)
3. The relationship may not be socially acceptable or legally sanctioned, as for an extramarital affair; unmarried or gender-nonconforming couples; or a nonbiological coparent.
4. The manner of death may evoke social stigma, as with HIV/AIDS or other contagious diseases. (For stigmatized loss associated with drug overdose or suicide, see Chapter 9.)

When circumstances surrounding a loss are hidden or involve highly charged social issues, the bereaved may suffer silently and in isolation. Lack of acknowledgment or stigma may lead survivors to minimize or distort their loss experience. If the family or community does not attend to and honor the loss, survivors may feel that their grief is inappropriate and they may be reluctant to ask for help. Further, the impact of a loss may be underestimated for certain family members, such as those living at a distance or estranged, or it might not be understood or have meaning for a small child or a loved one with cognitive impairment. Cultural modes of grieving that don't fit predominant social norms may be unacceptable or pathologized, such as traditional rituals or the wailing of mourners.

Social pressures can evoke shame, embarrassment, or fear of ostracism, inhibiting the bereaved from talking about highly charged losses and contributing to secret-keeping and distortion. Family members may collude to maintain painful secrets at great cost to physical and mental health (Imber-Black, 1993). Communication can become stilted or shut down completely, and members may avoid contact with one another and with friends, coworkers, or community members, increasing isolation. These patterns may become entrenched across generations, contributing to family myths about a loss. Without social or familial acknowledgment of significant losses, the bereaved can become blocked from expressing and integrating the loss.

Pregnancy Losses

Pregnancy loss in a miscarriage or stillbirth is often socially unacknowledged and minimized. Most prospective parents anticipate a successful pregnancy and bond early with the developing fetus. Both physical and emotional connections can make a pregnancy loss devastating. Many feel isolated, depressed, guilty, or angry and don't receive needed support. For couples, loving partners often grieve silently and separately. For single expectant parents, experiencing the loss on their own can be especially isolating.

When the loss of a pregnancy occurs, many are surprised at the intensity of their grief and feel others do not understand. Major sources of pain are in relinquishing hopes, expectations, and fantasies for the future of the child, anticipated parenting, and family life. With an eagerly awaited first son, daughter, or grandchild in a family, the loss is keenly felt in the kin network.

Miscarriage rates are rising now that a greater number of persons are delaying childbirth. Rates are highest for those with medical risks and with lack of access to good prenatal healthcare, particularly for low-income women of color. While miscarriage risks are multivariate, some expectant parents blame themselves or their partners, attributing their loss to poor diet, drinking, or stress.

Most miscarriages occur within the first 20 weeks and are unrecognized by others. Many women hesitate to share news of an early pregnancy or the loss and miss the support common after a child's death. As one woman remarked, "With a death in the family, there would be rituals to share that loss. If I'd had a serious illness, I'd receive get-well wishes and concern about how I was doing. For a miscarriage, there is none of that—just expecting me to bounce back to what's supposed to be normal life." Another woman recounted, "I tried to be OK around everyone. Just put it behind me and be chipper. The few people who knew didn't know what to say. So, nobody said anything." Grief can be more painful in contact with others who are excited over their pregnancies or newborns. One client related her painful experience a month after her miscarriage, when she was invited to a gathering to celebrate a new baby in her husband's family. "It didn't occur to anyone that it might be upsetting for me. I stuffed my feelings, got dressed up, and acted as if nothing was wrong. I can't forgive my husband for being so inconsiderate. Our marriage hasn't been the same."

It's important to explore the varied meanings of pregnancy loss in each experience. One mother felt guilty that she was more relieved than sad: she and her partner were already raising three children, one with special needs, and family life was highly stressful. For those who postponed childrearing, self-blame can add to anguish at a pregnancy loss. As one woman recounted, "We waited too long; I never pressed the issue and now, after two miscarriages, it seems too late." In a couple session, her partner acknowledged his part: "I didn't feel ready to raise a kid, so I just put it off—I'm so sorry we didn't have those important conversations."

In expectant couples, both partners are affected by the loss, yet many don't share their grief. Some dampen their own feelings to support their partner. As one woman reported, "I felt so alone. My husband seemed desperate for reassurance that I would be OK, so I pulled myself together around him. The only time I let myself cry was in the shower." Couple sessions can be helpful to normalize common gender differences in the loss experience. Miscarriage and stillbirth are physically and emotionally painful for women; sleep disturbances and irritability are common, with shock, disbelief, and intrusive thoughts. Sexual intimacy may be affected by strong hormonal changes, an induced termination or complicated birth, and associations of intercourse with the pregnancy and loss.

Marlene came for counseling 2 months after her miscarriage. "Nick and I had just shared our joy with everyone, so it felt especially cruel. Since then, I've been struggling and can't get motivated. I feel exhausted; some days I don't even want to get out of bed. Nick has been distant. I worry: Is he upset with me? I don't want sex. Does he blame me? Did I do something wrong? How do I bear up under this sadness?"

The therapist validated Marlene's experience of exhaustion, noting that her body and emotions needed time to adjust to what she'd been through. In a couple session, as Nick better understood her physical and emotional challenges and blame concerns, he was tender and reassuring. He acknowledged that he was hurting too, but he "stuffed it" so he wouldn't burden her and so he could keep up with heavy job pressures.

Prenatal Screening and Pregnancy Complications

Couple consultation is important when prenatal screening reveals a potential life-threatening situation for the mother or baby. Parents in shock and crisis need help to process the information. When a genetic disorder is diagnosed, anxiety, guilt, or shame commonly arise, as partners blame themselves or each other (or their family) for an inherited condition (Rolland, 2018). In high-risk pregnancies, clinicians can validate and normalize concerns and mood fluctuations; help them process information and options; and come to terms with a poor prognosis and altered dreams and expectations. In later pregnancy, induction of labor in giving birth to a nonliving fetus is physically and emotionally taxing, and sadness is profound.

Decisions to Terminate a Pregnancy

Decisions to end a pregnancy vary, in a range of circumstances, and are fraught with legal, social, and religious ramifications. If a serious, untreatable, or likely fatal abnormality is diagnosed, or if the pregnant woman's survival is at risk, time-sensitive considerations about terminating a desired pregnancy arise. The decision is often accompanied by profound depression and disorientation, and many avoid telling others. Elective termination is complicated by recent prohibitive laws, and miscarriage care may be denied by doctors, hospitals, and pharmacists.

Abortion is a highly stigmatized, unspeakable loss, usually kept private—even from one's partner or family. Most women who seek abortions are married, have one or more children, and are facing financial insecurity; others are young and single, many without a responsible partner. Most women experience relief after an abortion, yet feelings of grief or remorse surface for some and also for partners in committed relationships. Over half of abortions now occur through physician-prescribed, self-administered medications that induce the abortion in privacy at home, with telemedicine care provided and very low health risks. Yet, potential legal consequences are posed for providers, the pregnant person, and those who assist them. Most persons seek abortion in the first trimester of pregnancy, yet they may be denied by sanctions based on religious convictions that prioritize the life of the fetus from conception.

In the current American context, with the recent enactment of stringent legal restrictions, many face insurmountable barriers to access to care, particularly those with financial and/or health concerns, and even survivors of rape or incest. The plight for pregnant underage girls is of particular concern. In desperation, some women resort to unsafe procedures, with potentially fatal complications. With legal barriers, stigma, shame, and guilt surrounding abortion, many lack the support of family and friends in making the decision and in the aftermath. In faith communities that view abortion as a sin, elective termination of a pregnancy for any reason can bring harsh judgment, evoking profound guilt, anger, and alienation. Understanding and support are vital. Many groups supporting reproductive rights are mobilizing to restore access to those in need of services. In prevention efforts, the role of sexual partners in unwanted pregnancies requires more attention and accountability.

Perinatal Loss

With perinatal loss, shortly before or after birth, most prospective parents have formed a concrete attachment, making physical and emotional space for the new child. Typically, they have felt the baby kicking, celebrated with baby showers and gifts, arranged the nursery, and prepared older children for a new sibling. Hospital chaplains can be especially helpful with a loss. It can be comforting to send an announcement of both the birth and the loss, hold a simple but meaningful memorial with close kin, and save mementos, such as a tiny footprint or a lock of hair.

Perinatal loss is an ambiguous loss for siblings. Parents have the dual challenge of attending to their own emotional upheaval and to their other children's needs and concerns. Not seeing the baby makes the death less real and understandable. In one family, the 4-year-old, hearing his parents tell neighbors that they lost their baby, feared they might "lose" him on outings. Eagerness for a baby brother or sister may commingle with pangs of jealousy at the fuss over preparations. One child worried that her tantrum, breaking a baby gift, could have caused the death. Extended kin support of siblings is especially helpful. It's important to acknowledge the grief of grandparents and to urge relatives not to minimize the experience in an upbeat focus on future possible pregnancies.

After a pregnancy loss, heightened concern about the viability of another baby is common. Withholding the news of another pregnancy can be more isolating. Repeated pregnancy losses are deeply upsetting, with rising concerns about future success. Prenatal screening and genetic risk assessment are especially important.

Ray and Barbara sought couple therapy for intense conflict in the seventh month of their second pregnancy. Initial attempts to focus on future visions for the new baby fell flat. In exploring the meaning of this pregnancy and their past experience, they recounted the devastating loss of their first baby at birth. They were now highly anxious that the worst would happen again. Their families told them to push that bad event out of their minds. Each worried silently, keeping up a cheerful front, with anxieties spilling over into arguments about arrangements for the baby's room. Barbara wanted everything in order, while Ray put off setting up the crib, which was still in a huge box at the door.

Exploring further their earlier pregnancy experience, they recalled their initial excitement with family and friends and the "perfect" pregnancy they had. Tears then flowed in describing the shattering loss on what should have been their happiest day. They recalled the hushed voices of the medical staff in the delivery room and their utter devastation in learning that the baby would not survive. In the following months, each partner had ruminated over those searing events, and each saw an individual therapist briefly, but they had never shared their pain. Now their unspoken fears blocked them from investing in the child soon to arrive.

Acknowledging their deep sorrow, the therapist shared her admiration for their love and courage in trying anew for a much-desired child. Their fear and distrust of their obstetrician's assurances that everything was normal were understandable, since their last pregnancy had been normal. Meeting with a genetic counselor clarified that the loss carried no heightened risk for this pregnancy. They were encouraged to let family and friends know how they could be more helpful, instead of showing their constant cheer. As the couple shared and integrated their past loss experience, they approached the impending birth in joyful anticipation, assembling the new crib together.

For couples wishing to have their own biological children, repeated difficulties in pregnancy efforts can be devastating loss, dashing their hopes and dreams. It tends to be a hidden loss, socially unacknowledged, rendering the experience more painful and isolating. Disappointing the elder generation's wish for grandchildren can further burden them. Grief is more complicated with repeated costly, unsuccessful fertility efforts, sometimes over several years. Withdrawal, self-blame, or mutual blame can erode couple bonds.

Lucas and Isabel came for couple therapy on the brink of divorce after 3 years of unsuccessful fertility treatments, worn out and their savings depleted. They had lost all interest in sex associated with regimens for reproduction and had withdrawn emotionally from one another. Our first joint session had little energy or connection, as if the life had gone out of their bond. Their work in couple therapy eased their grief and revitalized their bond.

Deaths in Early Infancy

Sudden infant death syndrome (SIDS), usually occurring between 2 and 6 months of age, is poorly understood. It is commonly thought that the baby, while asleep, died of suffocation or choking or had an unsuspected illness. Several factors complicate this loss situation: The suddenness of the death is shocking, occurring without warning in babies that appear healthy. Ambiguity about the cause fuels suspicions about parental or care-giver negligence. The involvement of the legal system in some cases entails intrusive investigation of possible child abuse or neglect. Couple counseling is highly recommended, as tensions between parents, with suspicions or accusations of blame and guilt, increase risks for the breakup of their relationship. Sharing their loss with other families who have gone through a similar experience helps to relieve concerns. (The National SIDS and Infant Death Program Support Center is a valuable resource.)

Unacknowledged Loss in Other Significant Relationships

Attention to the bereaved is typically focused on the immediate family and often underestimates the significance of losses in the meaningful bonds in extended kin and social networks and other important relationships developed over the life course with close friends, companions, coworkers, mentors, long-term caregivers, and others. One who is grieving may be uncertain about expressing their feelings openly or may fear being inap-propriate or disrespectful to the immediate family. Often, their needs are simply lost in the overwhelming grief and preoccupation of those most closely affected.

Tara, age 38, married, with a teenage daughter, sought therapy for her-self, troubled by repeated upsetting dreams about her cousin, Allie, each time awakening with intense sobbing. Allie had died in a boat accident when they were at camp together at age 14. Tara had not gone on the boat ride. Events were a blur: She went home to the funeral, and her parents sent her right back to camp to help her get back to normal. Returning to camp, she had to sleep every night with her cousin's empty bunk above her. The camp held a fireside remembrance the first night, and then no one said anything more about the death or asked about her grief. (She now thought the camp minimized the accident so that they wouldn't be sued or lose campers due to families' safety concerns.)

Tara didn't remember grieving at all. Going home at summer's end, no one asked her how she was doing. Her mother was preoccupied in supporting Allie's mother, her mother's sister and Tara's aunt, who was devastated by the loss. After high school, Tara moved far away from her family and remained emotionally distant over the years. She went on with her life, putting the tragedy behind her, until now: having a teenage daughter brought it all back.

We began attending to Tara's long-suppressed grief, complicated by surviving Allie's death at camp and unsupported by her family and by the camp. I suggested she start journaling her childhood memories of Allie, their close bond, and their family life. Tara was especially upset with her own mother—"How could she have *not* understood what losing Allie meant to me? We were so close—we were born the same year, so they dressed us alike as babies. Allie was my best friend through childhood. We did everything together—except that fatal boat ride."

It is important to understand the profound and unique meaning of friendships and the breadth of emotions experienced when a friend dies. A close friend may provide a link to shared passions or pursuits, a common history or heritage, or ethnic ties and identity lost through migration. Friends often share similar beliefs and values and serve numerous social and emotional functions. They may help us develop a sense of belonging and community, increase our confidence, and share intimate and private communication. Friends frequently offer unconditional acceptance, give invaluable feedback, and allow individuals to fully "be themselves." While family relationships can serve similar functions, friendships are distinct in that they are usually chosen and are actively maintained because they enhance our lives. When a close friend dies, we lose both the friend and all that the friendship has provided.

As with family bonds, the closer and longer the friendship, the more profound the loss. With the loss of a kindred spirit or companion through life, many feel like they have lost a part of themselves. As one woman related, "Jenny knew me through two marriages and divorces and was always the one I could count on to understand and support me—more than anyone in my family." In conflicted or estranged friendships, grief can be complicated by a mix of sadness with anger, hurt, or remorse.

Friendship bonds are highly significant over the life course. For children and adolescents, close friends and peer groups are important in their social and emotional lives. The loss of a classmate or a teammate or coach touches all involved. Having a best friend or confidante can hold important meaning. The loss of a friendship that has buffered peer bullying or rejection, or a parental death or divorce, severs a vital lifeline for support; and it can reevoke the pain of the other losses. Clinicians can help parents understand children's grief and coach parents in having developmentally sensitive conversations and support (see Chapter 6).

For teenagers and young adults, the death of a peer—which is so out of sync with life-cycle expectations—evokes shock and disbelief that someone their own age can die, and they grapple to make sense of it and of their own vulnerability, particularly with a sudden or violent death (see Chapter 9). It's important to help them integrate the loss and hold a special place in their lives for the deceased. In midlife and later years, the deeply felt loss of a lifelong or childhood friend is irreplaceable. The loss of a neighbor or a companion for single, divorced, or widowed adults is often underappreciated, especially when family members do not live nearby, are estranged, or have died.

Death and Loss in School, Work, and Other Significant Groups

The impact of a student death ripples throughout the school community (see Chapter 9). Faculty and counselors are encouraged to hold group sessions with students, where all can come together, clarify information surrounding the death, express reactions, gain mutual support, and normalize any needs for grief counseling. Follow-up is important, since many students may initially be in shock, especially if a death was sudden and occurred in traumatic circumstances. Memorial services and plans to honor the memory of the deceased through positive action can foster personal healing, strengthen the community, and benefit others.

In adulthood, close bonds are often formed in the workplace. The death of a coworker or colleague can be emotionally distressing as well as disruptive to the daily routine and workplace functioning. Others may be unaware of the importance of the relationships for those who worked closely or felt a special rapport. Some may avoid or minimize their own sense of loss, particularly in a work culture that expects them to keep being productive. They must continue to function while constantly reminded of their loss, as they assume the duties of the deceased or glance at an empty desk or office.

The loss of a valued manager or employee may bring unexpectedly strong individual and collective grief, especially when there is strong group solidarity.

Tom, the foreman of a small construction company, stopped by to see me, saying he didn't need therapy but wanted to talk, knowing I worked with loss. He said he was "broken up" when one of his crew died, unexpectedly, of a heart attack. The company owner had quickly hired a replacement and was pressing the crew to complete a job, but they were arguing and making costly mistakes.

I asked Tom to tell me more about the worker who had died. His voice shook: "Clint was my right-hand man—I could always count on him. The replacement will be OK, but it won't be *him*. It won't ever be the same on our crew. I didn't realize he meant so much to me—and to all of us. We were like family." The crew had worked together for many years. We talked more about the strong bond among the workers and Clint's unique contribution. I encouraged Tom to meet with his crew to share how much Clint meant to them and how they missed him, and to find ways to honor his memory. They decided to donate their services as a crew to the local senior housing service where he had volunteered to complete the building project he had worked on. Clint's family gave Tom his toolbox, and he invited each crew member to keep one of the tools to remember him.

Those who are in supervisory, management, and caregiving positions, especially in educational, healthcare, and other professional settings, deal with their own grief reactions while helping others for whom they are responsible. Their own needs may go unacknowledged and unattended, while they are expected to perform their professional duties and care for others who look to them for strength and support. Managers, teachers, and helping professionals may stifle their own loss issues, including concerns about their possible role in contributing to, or failing to prevent, the death of a worker, student, or patient/client. Loss in a mentoring relationship is especially poignant. One teacher was devastated at the shooting death of a student with a promising future, whom she had mentored for several years. The death of a senior colleague, teacher, or coach is also keenly felt by those whom they mentored and inspired.

The grief of medical, mental health, and professional caregivers at the loss of a patient is often unacknowledged because they are trained to maintain some degree of professional detachment and because dealing with life-threatening conditions and loss is seen as part of their work (see Chapter 12). Grief can be especially strong for caregivers who have worked a long time and have developed a close bond with a person with special needs or chronic conditions. For those caring for the dying and for surviving loved ones, compassion fatigue is common, especially for bereavement counselors, hospital and military chaplains, and those working in oncology, nursing home, and hospice settings. In addition, they commonly question whether there may have been something more they could have done to alleviate suffering.

With a significant death, clinicians can support grieving staff, validate the meaning and importance of the loss, and encourage them to discuss it with trusted others in their workplace, kin, and social network. It is also important to work with educational, workplace, and healthcare systems to attend to the ripple effects of a death and loss in a school or work setting. Despite deadlines and the responsibilities that are to be carried on, all who are affected by the loss need time and support for mourning and adaptation.

Death of a Former Spouse

Grief at the death of a former spouse is unexpected and underappreciated by others. Mourning is complicated by the lack of social support and ambiguity in postdivorce attachments: their couple bond and intact family unit have ended, but both partners have gone on to their separate lives, often coparenting their children. It is natural, yet confusing, to feel deep sorrow that the person one once loved and shared life with has died, especially if the death is untimely or has occurred in tragic circumstances. Many ex-spouses get along well and often remain present in each other's lives. Many relationships continue to evolve in raising children. Grief reactions, while varied, can be more intense after a long marriage. They can reactivate strong emotions from the end of the relationship, particularly in highly contentious breakups, when grievances were not reconciled and with ongoing conflicts in childrearing.

Few social norms guide interactions or expectations for mourning. In social networks, some react with astonishment: "Why do you care? It was good riddance when he/she left you!" or "You left him! How could you be so sad!" Feeling pressed to explain the context of the divorce can reopen old wounds. With relational changes over time, such as remarriage, or with estrangement from former in-laws, one may not feel welcome to attend a funeral or memorial service, increasing one's isolation in grief.

> Janine, divorced for 12 years, was long out of touch with Sam, her former husband. Married in their graduate school years, they had had no children together. Sam had remarried and had two young children. An unexpected call from past neighbors informed her that Sam had died, at age 48, of a rare blood condition. Janine, in shock and feeling dizzy, went to bed. The next day she had a high fever. and her whole body ached. She could not get out of bed for several days, with intense flu-like symptoms. She wanted to offer condolences to Sam's family—she had been close to his parents. But she didn't want to intrude on his wife's grief (they had never met), and his children didn't even know he had been previously

married. At a later memorial event, she sat alone in the back row, silently holding in unexpectedly deep grief.

Janine met a few days later with a therapist, who helped her to unpack her complex emotions and sense of isolation in her grief. The therapist asked if there might be an old friend of the couple with whom she kept contact and who might share her grief. She called Alan, who spent a day with her, shared reminiscences, and took her to the grove of trees where Sam's ashes had been scattered. It was enormously healing for Janine, and she wrote a letter of condolences to Sam's parents, enclosing old photos of Sam she thought they would appreciate, and keeping copies for herself.

It's important for therapists to normalize strong grief as understandable given the past attachment and any ongoing coparenting relationship or friendship, and despite understandable reasons for divorce. Complicated feelings often surface from a painful or bitter divorce. A grieving former spouse can be encouraged to review the history of their marriage and divorce, remembering the love that was once there as well as any lingering regrets, conflicts, anger, or guilt.

When there are children from the past relationship, attention is also needed to their grief reactions, which tend to be complex. The death may reactivate feelings of abandonment by an uninvolved noncustodial parent, or it may reopen questions or pain surrounding the earlier family breakup. For some, the death dashes any lingering hopes of reunion, which are common for children after divorce. Any financial issues, such as child support or future needs, should be considered. Clinicians can encourage outreach to family members or friends to help all with this hidden loss.

Remarried individuals may constrain their grief so as not to upset their current partner or arouse their jealousy when they themselves are confused by the intensity of their grief. Strong grief reactions do not necessarily mean they are still in love with the ex-spouse, regret the past divorce, or do not love the current partner. Open couple communication is important, clarifying misunderstandings and strengthening a supportive bond.

Stigmatized Losses

Stigmatized losses stoke anxiety and defensiveness. They may be unmentioned or covered up to shield individuals and their families from shame, blame, or guilt, or from public or religious censure. Social nonacceptance of a relationship, as for LGBTQI+ persons, or stigma concerning the cause of death are particularly difficult for survivors.

Loss of a Hidden Intimate Relationship

Mourning may be complicated if a significant relationship is hidden from others, as with the death of a current or past secret lover. The exposure of an extramarital affair can be very painful and disrespectful for a grieving spouse and family and produce harsh social condemnation. If energy is consumed in hiding an intimate bond and covering grief, relationships with others may become strained or distanced, further isolating the bereaved.

Loss Complications in Gender-Variant Couples

For LGBTQI+ persons, mourning the loss of a loved one is particularly difficult in families and communities where gender-nonconforming identity and sexual orientation carry harsh social stigma or religious condemnation. While same-sex marriage is now legally sanctioned in the United States, many gender-variant couples and parents raising children continue to face painful stigma and harsh disapproval. The lack of social recognition or outright ostracism complicates their grieving process. Exclusion from funeral and burial rites by the partner's biological family or faith community denies the opportunity to participate in healing rituals and receive support. Partners who have not been public with their gender identity or sexual orientation may encounter more difficulty, especially those who lack a support system. In work settings and in heterosexual communities, their relationship may be hidden and relegated to the status of a bereaved friend.

The death of a life partner in older couples may also entail the loss of one's relational identity, which was often forged in overcoming many personal, familial, and social barriers. In conservative families and communities, it may arouse highly charged emotions in countering homophobia and establishing a marginalized sexual identity. Religious convictions opposing gay unions—love the sinner but condemn the sin—may compound grief and alienation. For older men, it can revive painful memories and guilt in having survived the HIV/AIDS epidemic in the gay community amid the many deaths of those near and dear to them.

Many bereaved spouses experience discrimination and disenfranchisement in medical and legal systems with the death of a partner or a nonbiological child. They may be denied visitation rights in hospitals, barred from medical decision making, and become ineligible to receive survivor benefits. Partners without legal rights to the body of the deceased cannot plan and execute their final wishes for burial or cremation. Some face legal challenges from biological family members. Where bereaved partners are excluded from formal mourning rites, it is crucial to create meaningful rituals that can include significant family members and friends. Families of choice, in extended friendship and informal kinship networks, provide essential supports in bereavement, especially for those facing nonacceptance from their families of origin.

When a couple has been raising children together, at the death of the biological parent the rights for custody and visitation by a nonbiological coparent may be denied or contested. In the United States, the varying state legal status of stepparent–child relationships renders a gay or transgender coparent legally vulnerable where existing policies (such as second-parent or joint adoption) are not accessible to them (Acosta, 2017). It is important to consult well-informed legal counsel. Advance planning is vital. Therapists can encourage discussion between partners, outlining in-the-event-of-death wishes in wills and communicating those decisions to extended family members. In cases where there has been ongoing involvement with a child by a surrogate or a biological parent from a former marriage, it's important to realign inclusive relationships for children's sense of security and well-being.

Stigmatized Cause of Death: HIV/AIDS and Other Contagious Diseases

The cause of death can be a source of stigma and disenfranchised loss, complicating mourning and adaptation. HIV/AIDS is the most stigmatized disease in recent times. Worldwide, the rates of infection and death steadily increased in low-income and ethnic/racial minority groups, affecting men, women, and children in utero. In high-risk regions, the deaths of men and women have orphaned children and taken a toll on extended families and communities.

With medical advances in prevention and treatment, persons can live with HIV as a life-threatening chronic condition. Yet, lack of access to costly, lifesaving drugs in underresourced communities, as well as the stigma attached to the virus, prevent many who are infected from receiving essential healthcare and social support, with increased risks for transmission and fatality. The cause of symptoms and death are commonly hidden, since those who disclose them face discrimination, rejection, or fear that survivors might infect others.

Social stigma also involves attributions of immorality and irresponsibility, since the risk of HIV/AIDS is associated with socially unacceptable practices, such as same-sex intercourse, promiscuity, and injection drug use. Those who contract HIV/AIDS are often blamed for bad lifestyle choices and are seen as deserving of their fate, in contrast to "innocent victims," such as children born with the virus and recipients of contaminated blood transfusions. In grappling with meaning making, a surviving partner exposed to similar risks may agonize, "Why him and not me?" Survivor guilt was common in the aftermath of the deadly HIV/AIDS epidemic in the 1980s–early 1990s that took so many lives in the gay community before effective treatments became available.

Deaths due to other highly infectious diseases also arouse fears of contagion and unsafe contact that could be fatal, as was the case with the Ebola virus and the COVID-19 pandemic (see Chapter 11). In some cases, family members cover up the cause of death to avoid social reproach and loss of support. Questions may imply judgment: "Was he vaccinated?"; "How did she get it?"; "Did anyone else catch it from them?" Such questions also arise from others' anxieties and attempts to reassure themselves that they are less at risk. Surviving loved ones may need guidance in navigating social stigma or blaming accusations.

Clinicians can help to normalize individual and family responses to stigmatized diseases, coaching parents on ways to talk about potentially fatal conditions with their children and others who are important to inform. Such conversations might include information regarding family members' health status, concerns about losing another caregiver or loved one, issues of discrimination, and general information about the disease and its treatment. Community forums and reliable web-based sites can be valuable in providing accurate information and countering unfounded fears and marginalization.

ATTENDING TO UNSPEAKABLE LOSSES

Grief processes are complicated in situations of ambiguous, unacknowledged, and stigmatized loss. The bereaved may minimize or block their own grief and suffer isolation without family and social support or culturally sanctioned rituals for mourning. Bereavement is hindered when a death is hidden or the significance of the loss is unrecognized. In many cases, the importance of the relationship and its loss are underestimated by others, or grief is considered inappropriate. The loss may carry the burden of shame and secrecy if the relationship is not socially acceptable, or the cause of death is stigmatized. Many of these issues arise in the loss of a cherished pet, to be addressed in Chapter 8, and in violent deaths, particularly with suicide, which is addressed in Chapter 9.

Meaning making is crucial to the grieving process. Bereavement is hindered not only by a lack of social support, but even more by social interactions or sanctions that undermine the mourner's attempt to validate and grieve their loss. Further, a spiritual crisis following bereavement may ensue from an unsupportive spiritual community. Clinicians are encouraged to explore the nature of the relationship lost and the meanings that it held for the bereaved. In addition, we should keep in mind that the grieving process is as personal and unique as the relationship itself; some will choose to express a great deal of emotion, whereas others may be more comfortable mourning the loss privately.

Clinicians can help the bereaved by validating the significance of their loss and fostering understanding of how such losses are marginalized. Grief work with families coping with unacknowledged or stigmatized losses should attend to members' varied experience, the family's shared understanding, and the broader sociocultural influences that impact the expression of their grief and the unhelpful response of others. Assessment should include an exploration of family legacies surrounding the meaning of illness, death, and grief, with special attention to family secrets, communication, and organizational patterns, as well as cultural, religious, and societal attitudes toward their loss situation. This can help clients in understanding the broader context in their mourning experience and in integrating their loss. Clinicians can encourage loved ones to seek out affirming communities and create meaningful rituals to mark the loss and honor the relationship. In experiences of empathic failure by important others, therapists might facilitate healing conversations.

CHAPTER 8

Loss of a Cherished Companion Animal

If there are no dogs in heaven, then when
I die, I want to go where they went.
—Will Rogers

Elza was surprised by the fullness of her grief after the sudden, unexpected death of Charlie, her canine companion for 10 years. In her journal, which helped her with her loss, she captured that strange, yet common, experience in grappling with the loss of a treasured pet.

There is a phantom dog in our house. I hear him breathing in his sleeping spot under our bed. I stretch my legs out gingerly on the sofa, so I won't disturb him. I reach down under the table as I'm eating to pet his fuzzy back. I spot the empty water bowl and think I must fill it. Taking off my shoes and dropping them on the floor I wince, thinking I might have hit him, lying in a favorite spot. On a trip downtown, I suddenly check my watch, thinking it's time to get back home, because the dog will be hungry.

The truth is, there is no dog in the house. There is only a pain where the dog once was, like the phantom pain of an amputated limb. A wisp, a breeze, a smell, a notion, a feeling, a void where the dog should be. I look around waiting to see this little bearded, black fluff ball, with the white blaze on his chest and his palm tree of a tail wagging in joy to let me know that today is the best day ever.

Elza later wrote:

The tests revealed a large mass on his spleen and internal hemorrhaging. Surgery wasn't advised because of high risks; the only decision left for us

146

was to euthanize him. Later that day, we returned to the clinic. and the vet brought Charlie to our car so we could say our good-byes. We called our son, Charlie's favorite person next to us, as we knew he would want to say good-bye, too.

We drove home broken-hearted and entered the house with a profound feeling of unreality. I slumped to the couch and felt I couldn't breathe. I stayed there the rest of the day. My husband and I have had alternating crying jags for weeks. We hold each other in deep grief. How could a small 12-pound dog have taken up such a prominent space in our house and in my heart? And now he is leaving phantom trails of himself everywhere.

THE RELATIONAL SIGNIFICANCE OF HUMAN-ANIMAL BONDS

The mental health field has been slow to recognize the significance of human–animal bonds and the loss of a companion animal (Walsh, 2009a, 2009b; Winch, 2018). Western philosophy and science have long held presumptions of anthropocentrism—asserting human uniqueness and superiority and regarding nonhuman animals as lower creatures, incapable of complex thinking or feeling. Such beliefs (which have contributed to inhumane treatment of animals) have influenced widespread assumptions that animal lovers merely misattribute "human" qualities and attachments to them. A large body of research now confirms that a wide range of species are sentient beings with remarkable cognitive, emotional, and social intelligence, albeit with differences related to their ecological niche. Most animals form strong social and emotional bonds within their groups and even across species, sustained through communication, collaboration, and mutual support.

Research on human–animal bonds has increasingly confirmed what pet lovers everywhere experience: the profound influence of dynamic relationships between people and their companion animals through their interactions and attachments (Fine & Beck, 2019). They provide many important physiological, psychological, and relational benefits contributing to well-being, healing from injury and loss, and resilience in facing adversity. They understand and communicate with their human companions in myriad ways. They relieve stress, provide pleasure and relaxation, and lighten moods. Dog walks provide exercise in nature and opportunities for social interaction. Offering deep affection and steadfast loyalty, these bonds bring joy and comfort.

At the heart of the relationship with pets is a unique affectionate bond. When well treated, they offer love, loyalty, and devotion that is unconditional, consistent, and nonjudgmental. In one study, women dog owners reported that unlike their human companions, they could count on their dogs to greet them enthusiastically on the worst days; not notice bad hair; forgive mistakes; and not need to talk things through. Some report that their pets provide the only uncomplicated relationship in their lives. Many experience a profound intimacy in this bond, enhanced through petting and cuddling, nonverbal communication, and sensory attunement of feeling states; studies confirm the positive physiological effects on neurotransmitters and the release of oxytocin.

In times of adversity, companion animals offer significant emotional support and meet relational needs for consistent, reliable bonds. They provide a sense of security and constancy, buffering transitions through disruptive life changes. As one woman related, "My cat, Minka, has been with me through two marriages, divorce, and widowhood as the one relationship I can always count on. I don't know how I'll carry on without her."

Pets are widely considered partners in life and valued members of the family. Human companions regard themselves as pet parents (rather than owners) in animal adoptions. Some raise a pet in preparation for—or in lieu of—rearing children. Their companionship is especially valued by children, the elderly, and persons living on their own. For many, these bonds also fill a yearning for closer connection with nature and other living beings. Some experience a deep affinity with animals that restores a sense of calm, balance, and harmony. As ancient Indigenous peoples have known, animals can teach us valuable lessons about life, from the natural rhythms over the life cycle to the joy in living and loving fully in the present.

IMPACT OF THE LOSS OF A COMPANION ANIMAL

Pets most often live their full lives with their human companions, and profound bereavement at their loss is normal and commonly as strong as for a significant human bond. Yet, the legacy of anthropocentrism often complicates bereavement with the loss of a companion animal.

Disenfranchised Grief in the Loss of a Pet

Despite their significance, attachment bonds with companion animals tend to be viewed as less important than human relationships. A lack of social acknowledgment and support with the loss of a cherished pet can complicate grief (see Chapter 7). Those who underestimate or trivialize the salience of the bond may respond dismissively: "Why are you so sad? It was only an animal." People who have lost their pets often feel pressure, even subtly, to justify the depth of their grief or the importance of their bond. As one client related, "I know some people think, 'Oh, it's just a dog. You can get another one.' Well, no. Roxi had her own personality and her own ways. She was always there for me and she loved me totally." The bereaved sometimes experience a disparaging response, such as "I could understand being so upset if it were a dog, but a bird?" One prominent professional woman, allergic to furry creatures, treasured her pet turtle, Tut, for over 20 years. When he died, close colleagues laughed at her tears, with mocking gestures of turtle hugs. She hid her grief and avoided contact with them for months.

The bereaved commonly feel embarrassed or even ashamed by how much sadness they're feeling, hesitating to disclose their feelings, sometimes even to loved ones. Their deep and unique bonds with companion animals may even be viewed as strange and their affections as pathologically misplaced. Strong attachments have been viewed as symptomatic of an unhealthy enmeshment or an inability to maintain healthy connections with humans. Studies suggest that feeling even closer to a pet than to other humans is not uncommon. The vast majority of pet lovers are not disturbed, socially inept, or trying to replace their human companions. Most people who connect strongly with animals also have a large capacity for love, empathy, and compassion. Most do not turn to pets as substitutes for failed interactions with humans. That said, individuals who have suffered relational abuse in human bonds and those who experience social stigma, bullying, or rejection, such as LGBTQI+ youth and those with intellectual differences, value all the more their trustworthy bonds and nonjudgmental acceptance.

Research finds that the strongly felt connections that people often report with their companion animals and the intensity of the relationships are similar to—and for some, stronger than—their human relationships. Studies applying attachment theory have found pets to be a consistent source of attachment security. Of note, compared with their relationships with romantic partners, individuals' attachments with pets were more secure on every measure. Another study, applying a self-psychology perspective, found that companion animals (including horses, dogs, cats, and rabbits) rivaled and even surpassed humans in their ability to provide important self-object needs, such as self-cohesion, self-esteem, calmness, soothing, and acceptance (Walsh, 2009a). It should not be surprising that the grief in losing a beloved pet can be just as strong—or even more so—as the grief suffered in losing a significant person in their lives.

Understanding the Meaning and Significance of the Loss

In light of the many varied roles that companion animals may play, it is crucial for therapists to understand the meaning and significance of the lost bond in each person's life. Not only does losing a pet create a significant void, but it also has ripple effects in disrupting meaningful activities, such as exercise and socialization in daily dog walks. Responsibilities in caring for a pet provide structure and meaning in daily life. Most missed are the emotional comfort and the playfulness, joy, and laughter a pet can provide.

For some people, bonds may be stronger because of hard times the human and animal companions have been through together. Seeking therapy several months after the death of her cat, one woman described her inconsolable grief: "Sunshine was my constant companion through my recurrent medical ordeals. She was my rock of stability and support." One widowed woman admitted, "To be honest, I think in grieving my dog, I have felt more deeply than I did losing my spouse." Another client reported, "When I lost my partner, there were many days I couldn't have gotten out of bed if Kato hadn't been there. He bounded on top of me to wake me, hungry and needing to go out. I had to take care of his needs— and he took care of mine through that dark year."

Some are surprised by the intensity and length of their grief process in losing a pet, making them aware of the significance of a bond that had been taken for granted. As one woman in counseling realized, "There was suddenly such an emptiness in my life." She shook off the impulse to quickly get another pet to fill the void. Beyond support for her grief experience, our meaning-making efforts focused on a wider appraisal of desired changes for more purpose and joy in her life and more satisfying human connections.

Companion animals can be a primary source of support for adults or children with special needs; their loss complicates coping abilities with life challenges. The death of a trained service animal is a profound loss for persons with serious physical or mental health challenges. These vital partnerships, usually lasting over the entire life of the animal, are essential in navigating everyday life and, for some, in preventing medical or psychological crises. Therapy and service animals provide essential support over many years for children and adults with developmental disabilities or serious mental and emotional health challenges. Persons who have survived harrowing trauma experiences, as in relational abuse or in military combat, may have a particularly difficult time coping with the loss of an emotional support animal that was vital in relieving anxiety, depression, or PTSD and in restoring a sense of connection, security, and well-being.

ADDRESSING PET LOSS IN COUPLES AND FAMILIES

Pets are well loved members in family life. Most often, they promote positive interactions; they can also become embroiled in relational tensions.

A systems perspective is important for understanding the varied roles animals play in couple and family functioning and the reverberations of pet loss in relational dynamics (Walsh, 2009b).

Pet Loss and Relational Dynamics in Couples and Families

When a pet has served a crucial function in couple or family dynamics, the loss of the animal can destabilize the relational system. Where couple or family tensions have been buffered by attention to—and from—a pet, their loss can increase relational distress and escalating conflicts. One woman's affectionate bond with her cat, Mitzi, compensated for a cool, distant relationship in her marriage. When Mitzi died, her husband's lack of affection became intolerable and she left him, just as some marital breakups occur when children have left home or when a child has died.

Complications can arise when companion animals become involved in ongoing relational dynamics, as in the following situation:

> Eric and Jack came to couple therapy on the verge of breaking up after 3 years together. Eric felt emotionally and physically neglected by Jack. Every evening, Jack would sit in his favorite chair, petting his cat Jasper on his lap, but he was emotionally unavailable and unaffectionate toward Eric.
>
> In exploring their connections, they both shared a love of animals; when they moved in together, they had adopted two cats—each partner enjoying a special bond with a favorite. Eric then choked up, remembering their first anniversary together, when his favorite cat, Simon, suddenly became ill, diagnosed with liver failure, and within days died in his arms. He grieved alone, aching for Jack's physical and emotional comfort in the loss. But Jack had distanced himself into his work, uncomfortable with Eric's strong emotions and avoiding his own grief. Since that time, it deeply pained Eric, sitting alone each evening, missing Simon, and watching Jack's affection toward his cat.
>
> Jack acknowledged that he had trouble showing affection with humans. He revealed, for the first time, that he had been sexually abused in his youth. He grew up taking care of wounded animals, feeling safe and emotionally nourished with them. Jack, a nurse, also had blamed himself for not having been able to save Simon's life. Eric listened and responded caringly. Both partners affirmed their deep love and desire to repair and deepen their bond toward a lifetime commitment.

Open Communication and Helping Children with Pet Loss

When families are constrained from talking about pet loss and sharing grief, it can stifle communication and block mourning. Some parents hesitate to openly discuss an impending or actual loss of a family pet with children, uncomfortable and uncertain about what to say. If they downplay a death to avoid their upset, children may feel embarrassed and alone in their grief and assume that the life and loss of an animal are unimportant.

Overall, children benefit from age-appropriate communication about animal loss to assist them through the grieving process (see Chapter 6). It's important not to assume that a child is too young to grieve. Families may need help to support their expressions of loss, and to not criticize tears or upset. It's also helpful when parents are honest and open about their own grief, or children may feel they should hide their reactions. It's important to give every family member a chance to work through their grief at their own pace.

Although some teenagers may minimize the importance of a pet and a small child or a family member with cognitive impairment may not fully comprehend a death, they may well have deep emotional ties and strong reactions to its loss. Sometimes, well-intentioned parents, wishing to protect young or vulnerable family members from upset, secretly remove a pet from the home without preparing them for the loss. As sad as it may be to anticipate the loss, it's more upsetting to find their pet suddenly gone and to miss a chance to hold it one last time. As appropriate, they should be offered a chance to say good-bye and can be encouraged to save a few treasured objects or toys and share active remembrances through stories and pictures.

In helping children with the death of a pet, it's important to be honest and clarify misunderstandings. Phrases such as "put to sleep" may imply that death is not final and can frighten them about what happens when they go to sleep. Simply saying that the pet went away leaves children worrying about where they went, what made them leave, and whether they will return. Children often blame themselves or fantasize worst-case scenarios. Imagining their pet lost, hungry, hurt, and in pain can bring more anguish than learning the truth. It's important to explain a pet's death sensitively, being clear that the pet will not come back but that it is free of pain or suffering.

The death of a pet, often the first loss that children experience, offers parents the opportunity to help them learn about love and loss and support their expression of grief. Two adult sisters recalled the time in childhood when kids had laughed at their tears when Toby, their hamster, died. Their father "made it better" when he comforted them and helped them bury Toby in a tiny box under a shade tree in their yard and share their memories of Toby. Parents should be prepared that a pet loss may arouse children's questions and concerns for discussions about death and the loss of human loved ones. Books, videos, and other resources for children can be helpful, yet the parents' own openness and availability for support matter the most.

The impact of loss for animals in the household should also be recognized. Clear signs of grief have been observed in many species, including domestic cats, primates, and elephants, with the death of a parent, offspring, or mate. Studies find that companion animals may show behaviors of profound grief with the loss of their human companions; some continue to wait or search for them. Moreover, pets in a household often form strong attachments to one another, even across species: surprisingly, dogs sometimes grieve for cats, and cats may even grieve for close canine companions. Surviving pets may withdraw, lose appetite and interests, and need extra attention. They may not readily accept a new pet in the home, but bonds typically grow with time.

COMPLEX AND TRAUMATIC CIRCUMSTANCES OF LOSS

The grief experience is influenced by the way the animal loss occurs. Grief can be more painful and bereavement more complicated in unexpected or traumatic circumstances, particularly with sudden and untimely loss; accidental death, negligence, or deliberate harm; ambiguous loss; and forced relinquishment. In some cases, grief is compounded by other losses. Considerations in euthanizing pets that are aged or suffering pose agonizing dilemmas for many pet lovers.

Sudden and Untimely Loss

The sudden and premature death of a pet is shocking. The bereaved lack time to prepare emotionally and to say their good-byes. For some, their surprising grief brings awareness of the significance of the bond lost.

> When her daughter moved to an apartment that didn't accept pets, Ursula took in her 4-year-old dog, Bailey, not expecting to become emotionally attached. Ursula, an artist who worked in her home studio, found Bailey a welcome companion, especially enjoying their daily walks in nearby woods. At age 8, Bailey died suddenly, after eating contaminated dog food. Shocked by the death, her intense upset and long-lasting grief caught her by surprise. She hadn't realized she had become so deeply attached.
>
> Living alone without family nearby, Ursula found solace in a handwritten letter and photos she received from her daughter. She wrote back: "It meant so much to me to receive your remembrances of Bailey,

romping on the beach. I've managed to distract myself with errands and projects, yet at odd moments I do let out a wail to fill up this empty house. Still, I want to remember him best by finding ways to incorporate his joie de vivre into my everyday life."

Accidental Death and Issues of Negligence or Abuse

A pet death due to an accident is traumatic and commonly provokes blame or guilt about responsibility (see Chapter 9). One father could not forgive himself for running over his children's beloved kitten when he hurriedly backed out of the driveway. A death involving negligence, compounded by minimization, can seriously strain relationships, as in the following case:

> When Marge and Herb came to therapy, she had been withdrawn and upset with him for months. Herb said she always seemed agitated, finding fault with everything he did. In exploring the situation, Marge related that 6 months earlier he had absentmindedly left her beloved terrier Fluffy in the car after a morning errand. When she arrived home from work at the end of the day, she was distressed that Fluffy was missing. Finding him dead in the car, she was distraught. To relieve her upset and to assuage his guilty feelings, he minimized the loss, assuring her that they could get another dog just like Fluffy. The next day he brought home a new puppy from a shelter. Outraged, she made him return the pup. She carried long-simmering fury at his carelessness and insensitivity to all that Fluffy had meant to her—Fluffy could not simply be replaced like a stuffed toy.

A pet death caused by deliberate harm is the most wrenching. Studies of domestic violence find that perpetrators of abuse often threaten to kill a cherished pet (see Chapter 9). A partner facing the threat or actual harm to pets often will stay in the abusive situation rather than abandon the pet when shelters for abuse survivors or other accommodations do not allow animals.

Ambiguous Loss

In situations of ambiguous loss, when the fate of a missing pet is unclear, various imagined scenarios of harm and suffering can be agonizing. Conflict between family members can arise, as some hold out hope of return while others come to accept the loss as final and want to grieve and move on. After a disappearance, some may be tormented by thoughts of what might have been done to prevent the tragedy.

In the turmoil of a widespread disaster, such as a wildfire or hurricane, when a pet is left behind or runs off, concern over its fate may be minimized by others who are contending with devastating losses in human lives, homes, and communities. Even so, many post pictures of the missing pet in the area or on the internet. Animal rescue groups rally in disaster situations to save stranded pets, arrange foster families, and strive to reunite them with their human companions.

Forced Relinquishment

One of the most agonizing situations is the forced relinquishment of a valued pet. Pets may be given up due to unsafe home conditions with concerns of pet abuse or neglect. When human companions face financial duress and/or housing insecurity, pets may not be accepted in shelters or new rental accommodations. Older adults, or those suffering serious illness or disability, may be forced to give up their cherished pet if they can no longer care for them or when they must move into a long-term residence or nursing home that does not allow animals.

Grief is compounded by concerns about the fate of a relinquished pet, especially for animals that are older or infirm and less likely to be adopted. If a cherished pet is given up to animal rescue services, the bereaved's sadness may be eased by hopes that the animal will be adopted. Yet most deal with ambiguous loss, uncertain of their pet's fate and well-being. Some carry long-term anguish, imagining that their pet might have faced neglect and death in a kill shelter, which is more common in low-income and rural communities. "No-kill" animal shelters and rescue agencies make every effort to find caring foster and adoptive homes for relinquished pets, but usually a bereaved human companion never learns their fate. It's important to attend to their concerns and whenever possible, support advance planning and efforts to assure that an animal will be well cared for.

In a natural disaster or a war zone, attachment to pets can be so strong that some are reluctant to leave their animals behind, even if staying with them endangers their own safety. Many, with great difficulty, take pets with them, only to be forced to separate later when authorities don't allow animals in public spaces, transportation, shelters, or across borders. Leaving a cherished pet behind to an uncertain fate can be unbearable, especially for children.

Concerns about abandonment or guardianship of pets come to the fore when their human companions are doing end-of-life planning. One elderly couple had deep concerns about the future well-being of their beloved parrot, Coco, expected to live many years after them. Old family conflicts were revived in arguments over which of the adult children could be trusted to provide the care they expected for Coco. A family consultation proved very helpful.

Grief Compounded by Other Losses

A pet loss amid other losses or disruptive transitions, as in divorce or migration, can have a cumulative impact, compounding the grief. One man learned that his dog, Buddy, had inoperable cancer shortly after his wife divorced him and his son had left home for college. The pileup of recent and anticipated losses was too much to bear. Sleep problems and heart palpitations led him to a medical consultation with his primary care doctor. Along with a thorough medical checkup, she listened attentively to his recent cascade of losses and referred him to a behavioral health therapist for help in addressing his grief.

When a pet has helped to ease the difficulties of hard times, its later loss can reactivate the past losses (see Chapter 10). If a pet has been a companion over many years, the bond and grief can be especially strong, and even more so when it revives emotions from other lost attachments.

> Roger grew up on a farm always wanting a horse, but his father had repeatedly refused. When he was 12, his mother developed cancer and urged her husband to grant Roger's wish. The devotion and affection Roger gave to and received from his horse, Sugar, helped him to cope with his mother's illness and then her death. Shortly after he left home for college at 18, his father casually mentioned in an email that he had sold the horse because caring for it was too much trouble. This abrupt news was devastating, and it also re-evoked the painful loss of his mother. His father's callous disregard for his feelings sparked an angry and long-lasting cutoff from him.
>
> In father–son telehealth therapy sessions, the father gained appreciation of Roger's meaningful bond with Sugar. He then tearfully acknowledged how much he missed his wife and his son and that the horse had been a constant painful reminder of both losses. He had thought that selling it would relieve his sadness, but it only left him feeling all alone. The mutual understanding and caring father and son gained through this therapeutic conversation brought them to a closer relationship than they had had in the past and Roger returned home often to visit.

End-of-Life Decision Making

Navigating end-of-life issues with a cherished pet is commonly painful and difficult. When a client's companion animal is ill, injured, or aged, it's important to have sensitive conversations with them about end-of-life considerations. As in human relationships, the death of an older animal is to be expected, yet the loss of a longtime companion can be profound. In families, ideally, a life-ending decision is made with the input of all members, including children as age appropriate. Regardless of the decision, children need to be informed in a sensitive way about both the potential death and what will happen once their animal dies.

Increasingly, persons who are strongly attached to their pet are electing costly, extensive medical treatments, unless the animal's suffering or the financial or caregiving burden is too great. These can be wrenching decisions, given the treatment risks, their high cost, and lack of affordable insurance coverage. Some will spend limited funds on their pet's treatments and medications, while cutting back on their own needs. The dilemmas need to be discussed sensitively, exploring any guilt at forgoing treatments, with a veterinarian, who can provide clear information about medical options and prognosis. In navigating end-of-life issues, animal hospice programs focus on extending a pet's quality of life. That might mean treating a seriously ill or frail pet "in kind and gentle ways" by supportive care like hand feeding or giving fluids, oxygen, or pain medication.

Pet lovers hope for a natural, peaceful death after a long life for their cherished companions. But this idealized scenario is often unrealistic and may not be easy, kind, or peaceful. Waiting for a natural death can prolong suffering, which is often unseen or minimized, since animals don't show their pain as humans might. A peaceful passage is more likely with veterinary consultation: to make a pet more comfortable when treatment is not advisable and to consider euthanasia.

Many people are uneasy even thinking about euthanasia. Physician-assisted dying is highly controversial in human end-of-life care, with profound ethical and religious considerations (see Chapter 4). This may be the first situation where individuals are called upon to make such a permanent and heartbreaking choice to end a life of a loved one. Yet, it has long been common practice to "put down" a frail animal or to drop off an infirm pet at the vet without participating in a life-ending decision. Studies find that in most cases, euthanasia is more beneficial for both the animal and human companions than waiting for a suffering pet to die "naturally."

In making critical end-of-life decisions, a veterinarian can best assess the animal's condition and prognosis. Yet, human companions may be best in assessing the quality of their pet's daily life and suffering, as well as their own needs and constraints. The physical demands, needs, and limitations of caregivers, and their situational constraints, as in lifting a heavy animal up and down stairs, all should be considered. A decision to end an animal's life may be recommended if the pet is in constant pain, if undergoing a highly stressful treatment ordeal would not likely help and could increase suffering, or if the pet is unresponsive to affection, unaware of surroundings, and uninterested in life.

In end-of-life decisions, there are likely questions or even personal turmoil about making the right choice about whether it is the appropriate time. Still, that choice can be painful. One woman shared her decision to end the life of her horse: "It was just agony to see this beautiful animal struggle in pain to walk and to be so helpless. I was distraught to lose him, but I would look into his eyes and see his suffering and know that the only humane choice was to end his pain."

Understandably, when pets have been deeply enmeshed in their humans' lives, those who love them want to hold on to them for as long as possible. In cases where pets' suffering is prolonged when their human companions are unable to bear losing them, it is important to understand their reluctance and help them weigh considerations. The decision might be seen as the final act of love that the human partner can make for their cherished animal. As one dog dad said, "I kept putting it off, even though I knew it was the best thing to do. But I realized it was unkind to keep him alive for my own needs when he was suffering so much. It was the hardest—yet most compassionate—thing I've ever done in my life. And I think the experience made me a kinder, more considerate person in all my relationships."

An emergency situation may prompt a life-ending decision. One couple later came to counseling agonizing over the sudden events: "Out of the blue, our precious cat, Juniper, started having convulsions and didn't recognize us or her surroundings. Our vet advised us that it was likely an inoperable brain tumor and recommended euthanizing. In our upset, we went ahead without time to process it and now we're second-guessing, 'Did we do the right thing?'" It was helpful to validate their conflicted emotions and support their decision as truly humane.

Increasingly, veterinarians offer the option to be present, either at the clinic or at home, and they play a comforting role during the procedure. Those who may not want to be present should be given the opportunity to say their good-byes in their own ways and to have their preference respected. Being present may be too distressing for young children or others, whose intense reactions could also upset the animal. Those who do wish to be with their pet at the end of life most usually find it a very healing experience. One couple found it enormously comforting to hold their cherished beagle in their arms as the veterinarian administered the sedating medication, followed by the lethal drug. They said that after experiencing his painless passing, they were wishing that when their time comes to leave this earth, they and their human loved ones could have such a loving and peaceful ending.

In matters of pet illness, end-of-life decisions, and bereavement, therapists are playing a collaborative role with veterinary specialists in clinical services or community education. Some veterinary settings now offer mental health services to clients to help those coping with natural and unexpected death, as well as the unique decisions and emotions concerning pet euthanasia.

Facilitating Grief and Fostering Healing and Resilience

Preparing for the anticipated loss of a valued animal companion can help clients in their grieving process. Clinicians can explore the impact of the loss and its influence on their quality of life. Normalizing a commonly minimized or stigmatized experience of loss is crucial, as is mobilizing resources to support grief. It is important to explore varied coping strategies in bereavement. In one couple, Jaime found it helpful to plunge right back into important work projects, while Boris couldn't focus on work and needed time off. They took long walks and quietly comforted each other. Initially, they avoided other contacts, since they just did not want to talk to anybody. After a few weeks, they found it easier to see and tell coworkers—and were surprised and moved by their caring response. "Both of us had a zillion pictures of Rocco on our desks—we laughed together realizing that we didn't have our own photos, only pictures of our dog! So, everybody at work knew Rocco."

Clinicians can be helpful in facilitating key adaptational tasks with the loss of a pet, as with human losses in the family (see Chapter 5), in the following ways:

1. Help the bereaved to clarify and share information, acknowledge the loss, and gain understanding of its meaning and significance for family members and relationships.

2. Facilitate open communication and shared experience of loss by encouraging healing rituals, expression of feelings, and kin and social support.

3. Facilitate discussion and efforts to realign daily life patterns and relationships disrupted by the loss.

4. Support reinvestment in other relationships and continuing bonds with the lost pet through stories, photos, and deeds of remembrance.

Meaning making is crucial in grieving the loss. It is important for therapists to learn about the unique qualities of the companion animal, the history and significance of relational bonds, and the meaning that its life and death have for those bereaved. Some interpret their experience in the context of their life course expectations and their comparisons to other loss events in their lives, especially in their human relationships. In couples and families, the attachment and loss may hold different meaning and value for spouses or various members. It's very important to acknowledge and normalize differences while encouraging the validation and empathic support of those who are most deeply affected. Besides sorrow and loss, more complicated reactions are not uncommon. Guilt and remorse may be aroused for persons feeling responsible for the pet's death, as for an accident that took its life. Anger may be strong in situations of negligence or forced separation.

Therapists should also attend to broader social and cultural influences in unhelpful responses of others and identify potential resources for healing. In fact, with animal rights awareness and pet adoptions increasingly widespread, social awareness and compassion in pet loss are becoming more common. For example, neighbors commonly rally to search for a missing pet. Support is frequently received in sympathy cards for pet loss, social media posts, and online companion animal networks. One man, in a posting to his neighborhood dog parents group, invited others to join him at the dog park for his dog's last visit before euthanasia.

It's most important to validate and normalize intense grief. It can reduce their worry that there is something wrong with them if they feel devastated by the loss of such a relationship. Therapists can help clients to appreciate that people experience their grief in different ways. As in the loss of a human bond, different facets of grief may emerge. Sadness and yearning for the pet and the companionship loss are most common. When it is difficult to accept that the pet is really gone, it's not uncommon to hear barking or scratching at the door or to expect the pet to greet you upon coming home. Besides sorrow and loss, it is not unusual to have more complicated feelings. Guilt and remorse may be aroused in those who feel responsible for the pet's death. Anger may be strong in situations of negligence. For those experiencing profound suffering, therapists should check that their basic needs in living are being met, as in asking about eating and sleeping habits, safety, shelter, and hygiene.

As is true of mourning a significant human loss, there is no right or wrong way or a certain length of time to grieve. It's important to encourage the bereaved to take the time they need to work through grief. Others often urge them to quickly get another pet to "get over" their loss. Some may want to get a new pet quickly, while others may feel reluctant or even disloyal. It's important that they feel ready and eager to build a new, loving relationship. Some may want to get a different breed, and others may want a similar animal, hoping for a familiar bond. The latter can lead to disappointment when the animal's temperament or attachment is not the same. Rather than thinking of the new animal as a replacement, it's important to foster each animal's development of its own personality and unique bonds.

Steps in Healing; Acts of Remembrance

Bereaved clients can be helped to expect and honor complex emotions in grief and to express mixed feelings to trusted family and friends. As they feel ready, it can be healing to talk with others about their pet, what the pet meant to them and what will be missed, and to reminisce about the good times. Sharing their experience may bring the recognition that all living things will die and that grief is both a unique and a universal experience.

Clinicians can encourage the bereaved to create healing rituals to mourn their loss and honor their companion animal (Imber-Black, 2012). Some find it helpful to express feelings and memories in a photo collage, poems, or stories. A simple memorial rite can be very healing, with family members or friends sharing favorite memories of their pet. Shared activities are especially beneficial in families, such as creating a photo album of their life with their pet. Many bury the remains or scatter the ashes in a special place they had enjoyed with their pet. Many donate to animal welfare organizations or shelters in their memory.

Many therapists have had deep connections with a childhood pet or recent companion animal, and have experienced the surprising depth and complexity of feelings with their passing. In my family of origin, painful losses were not talked about (see Chapter 12). So it was not surprising that one day I came home from school and my parents said simply that our aging dog Rusty, my constant companion, had died. They didn't say how. I suspected they had taken her to the vet to end her life, since we were moving to California a month later. But I never asked, and we each kept our grief to ourselves.

Times have changed. In family life with my husband and daughter, we have loved and lost two wonderful dogs. I share here, our recent experience:

> I continue to miss our beloved dog, Shasta, a joyful Lab–Golden mix that we lost at age 14, over 2 years ago. When she first had seizures at age 12, we, and our vet, began to anticipate that we might not have her with us much longer. We weren't ready to hear that. But we were fortunate: medication controlled her seizures, and she lived a healthy, happy life for another 2 years, until a progressive neurodegenerative condition and other infirmities took a toll.

Like other pet lovers, I hoped she might die peacefully in her sleep when the time came (and many days, as she was sleeping, I'd come close to hear if she was still breathing). Yet, her appetite and joyful spirit remained strong, and she enjoyed "stroll and sniff" walks every day. Sometimes, she would lose her balance and fall over, yet she'd lie there, smiling up at me, as if to say, "I'm OK, and it's nice here, lying in the grass; let's just stay awhile." And we did. Then I'd help her up and, rallying, she'd want to go farther. For me, our daily strolls became my walking meditation: being fully present in the moment in nature and vicariously enjoying her sheer pleasure, seeing a squirrel but no longer caring if she chased it.

Amazingly, when summer came, Shasta was able to make one last trip with us to our vacation cottage. She could no longer run on the beach or swim, but she delightedly splashed and soaked in the plastic kiddy pool. As her condition worsened and her struggles increased, we had family discussions with our vet to decide when would be the compassionate time to end her life. We were with her for that final hour with our vet. We held her and comforted her as she was sedated and gently went to sleep. We—and our vet—were tearful after saying our goodbyes to her. Yet we felt grateful for all the time we were fortunate to have her with us, so loving and joyful. Remembering the jar of treats she had loved at our vet's office, I thanked the staff for their care by sending *them* a giant box of chocolate treats.

After losing Shasta, I missed my constant companion, and the house seemed empty without her physical presence. I found comfort and a sense of connection in setting her vial of ashes on a bookshelf, along with a favorite photo, dried flowers, a candle, and a small Inuit sculptured bear. Over several weeks, I sorted through hundreds of photos taken over the years, compiling and sharing a photo scrapbook of our favorite family times together. It was consoling to receive caring messages and calls from extended family and friends. We plan next summer to scatter her ashes at the water's edge of the shore where she loved to chase the birds.

CHAPTER 9

Violent and Traumatic Deaths

Fatal Accident, Homicide, Overdose, Suicide

> To lose our son in such a violent way was unimaginable.
> Our family is torn apart. We'll never be the same.
> —A Bereaved Parent

The loss of a loved one in traumatic death circumstances can wound the body, mind, and spirit of survivors and can shatter family bonds, as in the following tragedy:

One father sought therapy after the death of his 22-year-old son, Nick. He had taken Nick and his brother, 28-year-old Cory, on a kayak trip in the Pacific Northwest. When a sudden violent storm erupted, Nick's kayak overturned, and the surging waters carried him over the rapids. His battered body was found the next day in the rocky shoals. The father and brother managed to keep their boats upright and survived.

The therapist met initially with both parents, who were distraught that their son's life was cut short in such a horrific way. After overcoming early childhood developmental challenges, Nick had just graduated from college and was excited about a new job. As they explored the family impact, the mother said, brusquely, that she had not been in favor of the trip; she believed kayaking in such rough waters was too dangerous. Now she was consumed in managing all the practical matters with the death and the outpouring of sympathies from their community. She said, "I don't have time for grief or therapy—anyway, my husband is the one who needs the help."

The father said he felt doubly guilty for Nick's death because this had long been his dream trip. He put his children in harm's way and was unable to save his son. He was very worried about Cory, who had survived that terrifying situation when his brother didn't. Cory had with-drawn into his work, avoiding family contact. The father added, "He's always needed order and predictability and was never one to express his feelings." Their other child, Luci, age 25, was pregnant, so had not gone on the trip. She was now keeping a lid on her grief, concerned that it might affect the pregnancy. The father lamented, "We're each adrift on our own lifeboats."

   The parents agreed on the need to come together to heal their fam-ily. Over the next 3 months, they all participated in combined individual, couple, and family sessions, coordinated by a team of systems-oriented therapists, sensitively attuned to separate and shared needs and concerns.

A systemic, resilience-oriented practice approach in violent and traumatic situations considers the multiple influences in the death and its aftershocks for all survivors and their bonds. It contextualizes the dis-tress, addresses the individual and relational impact, and strengthens fam-ily capacities for both individual and collective recovery and resilience (see also Chapter 11).

TRAUMATIC LOSS IN FAMILIES: AN UNTHINKABLE TRAGEDY

Deaths in violent and traumatic circumstances are shattering in family life, affecting all members, their bonds, and the family unit; they pose risks not only for individual dysfunction but also for relational conflicts and family breakdown. The experiences of trauma, loss, and grief are intermingled. Symptoms such as depression, anxiety, substance abuse, and relational conflict or withdrawal are common. Surviving loved ones blocked from healing may perpetuate wider suffering through self-destructive behavior or suicide or in taking revenge toward others. Massive ongoing or histori-cal trauma, with loss of hope and positive vision, can fuel transmission of negative transgenerational patterns (see Chapters 11 and 12). With brutal atrocities and injustice, the impetus to restore a sense of family or commu-nity honor can either fuel cycles of retaliation or spark courageous efforts to rise above the tragedy.

   Initially, the surviving loved ones are overwhelmed. Those reeling from the news commonly react differently, with emotions ranging from numbness and disbelief to intense and unbearable pain. Most experience a dizzying sense of disequilibrium. In neurophysiological effects, a trau-matic loss experience floods the brain with neurotransmitters, and the central nervous system becomes highly stimulated. Some feel as if they have been "hit in the gut," their stomach churning or in knots. Some can't concentrate or face the loss; others can't stop thinking about what has happened. Others have trouble sleeping—or want to sleep all the time. Still others have no appetite, while others are insatiably hungry. Some lose all desire for sex, while others crave sexual intimacy. Some can't focus on anything except the tragedy, repeatedly questioning how it could have happened. Often, they agonize over how they—or others—could have prevented the terrible death.

The impact can be especially strong for those who were present and witnessed the death, for those who may have barely survived themselves, or for those who blame themselves for the tragedy. Many are plagued with self-recriminations or mutual blame, which can fuel relational conflict or estrangement. Some become trapped in a victim position, blaming others, and blocked from healing and growth by anger or wishes for revenge. For some, grieving may be so intense and overwhelming they are unable to function, which could lead to additional losses of job and financial security. Some lose a sense of identity or purpose. Conflict or withdrawal in couple and family relationships is common.

Traumatic grief is most common when deaths are sudden, violent, and untimely. It is especially cruel when the loss upends the "natural order" of generational life passage with the death of a child, even in young adulthood. Yet, while elders are expected to die in later life, a death may be untimely, as at retirement, shattering hopes and dreams on the brink of a new life phase:

> Kamara and her siblings were in anguish over the sudden, tragic deaths of their parents. After working tirelessly at physically demanding jobs and raising their children lovingly, they had looked forward to a leisurely retirement. As the parents drove to their new home in Florida, an oncoming truck swerved across the highway median, hitting them head-on. The family was inconsolable: "They saved up and dreamed about this time of life; they sacrificed so much for us and deserved to enjoy their golden years! It's so unjust!"

Accidental Deaths: Negligence, Blame, Accountability

Because parents are responsible for the safety and well-being of their children, their grief can be compounded by agonizing questions of their negligence in the accidental death of their child.

> After the long pandemic winter, Gina and Doug, excited for a weeklong summer vacation with their three young children, rented a house with a swimming pool in the countryside. On the last morning, as the parents were packing up to go home, their 3-year-old son wandered into the

kitchen and pushed open the screen door into the yard. The parents, searching for him, found his lifeless body at the bottom of the pool. They were unable to revive him. The emergency medical technicians rushed him to the nearest hospital. Although there was no brain activity, he was kept on a ventilator for 7 weeks, prolonging the parents' agony. (By that state's law, life support could not be removed until there were no longer any physical reflexes.)

The parents were torn apart in their anguish. Doug became consumed in legal actions to sue the rental agency and the homeowners for failing to provide a cover for the pool. Simmering beneath the surface were their mutual accusations and self-blame for losing sight of their toddler in their haste. They came to therapy 9 months later, as their marriage was crumbling. Their surviving son, age 7, was misbehaving, and their daughter, age 5, was having night terrors and clinging to her mother.

In therapy, it's crucial to explore beliefs and accusations about blame and guilt that complicate bereavement. It's helpful to acknowledge common concerns and human limitations in control, while also examining accountability for actions or inactions that might have contributed to the tragedy.

Multistressed families, overloaded with concerns, are at higher risk of a tragic accident. A single parent is readily subject to presumptions of fault.

One morning, Tanya, a single parent, had to take her 6-year-old daughter, suffering a painful earache, first to a doctor's appointment and then to school before going to her job. Her boyfriend, Chris, who had spent the night, offered to drop off her younger child at the daycare center on his way to work. Delayed in traffic and preoccupied with financial worries, he drove straight to his job, completely forgetting about the sleeping boy in the back seat of his car. Tanya went to pick up her son at day care in the afternoon, soon learning he had never arrived. The provider had left a voice message, asking about him, which, in her hectic workday, she had not yet picked up. She called Chris, who rushed to his car, finding the boy's limp body. He apologized profusely, but Tanya, devastated by the death, was furious at him. Escalating conflict led the couple to break up. Tanya's parents blamed her for trusting Chris, and she berated herself. Police and legal involvement intensified the situation.

When an accidental death is caused by reckless actions or negligence, criminal charges may be brought. Loved ones seeking justice may be embroiled over months or years in agonizing legal battles that further complicate and prolong grief.

When a Loved One Is Killed

The term *homicide* refers to a range of acts that cause another person's death. Here we consider the impact for survivors and their relational systems when a loved one is killed. In one family, the death of the oldest son, age 17, in a shooting was most devastating for the youngest son, age 8, who looked up to his big brother like his "second dad." Several times he ran into the street wanting a car to hit him so he could die to be with his brother.

Family Impact of Violent Deaths

The shock and pain of a tragic killing can shatter family cohesion, leaving members isolated and unsupported in their grief. When grieving is blocked, emotions may explode in conflict; some children internalize their grief in symptoms of anxiety or depression, while others externalize their distress in behavioral problems. Adolescents may withdraw from the family and/or engage in risky behavior and drug or alcohol use. Unbearable feelings may be expressed in a fragmented fashion by various family members. Often, therapy is sought for a child's problems that are related to the loss, but without mention of the death, as in the following case (in Walsh, 2016c):

> Referred by a school counselor, Mrs. Ramirez sought help at the child guidance clinic for her 11-year-old daughter Teresa's school problems over recent months. In the first session, the therapist and mother focused on Teresa, who seemed listless and at a loss to explain her inattentiveness and the drop in her grades. The therapist initially focused on parenting skills to support Teresa's mood and studies, with no improvement. Invited as a consultant, I suggested exploring recent stress events in the family as a potential source of concern. Four months earlier, the oldest son, Miguel, age 18, had been hit by a stray bullet in gang crossfire. The shot that killed him had also shattered the family cohesion. The father withdrew, drinking heavily to ease his pain. The second son carried the family outrage into the streets, seeking revenge for the senseless killing. A younger son was quietly keeping out of the way. Mrs. Ramirez, alone in her grief, deflected her attention to Teresa's school problems (see Figure 9.1).
>
> Family sessions provided a context for shared grief work. It was especially important to involve the younger brother, who the mother said was behaving "as good as gold." He had been holding in his own pain at losing his brother so as not to further burden her. He also shared his worries for his own safety, coming of age as a young male of color, with ongoing threats of violence, gangs, and drugs in the neighborhood.

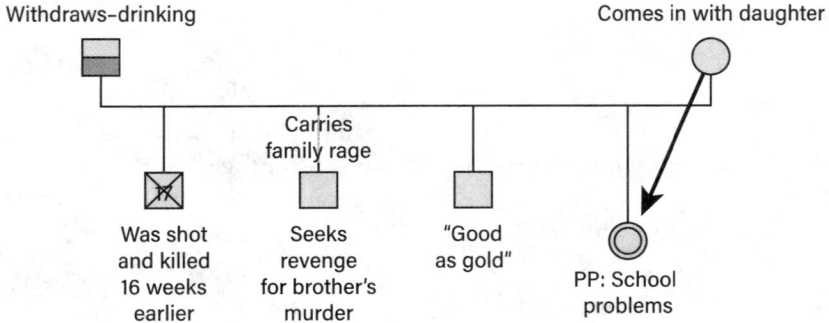

FIGURE 9.1. Genogram highlighting the impact on the family system of the traumatic death of the oldest son. From Walsh (2016b). Copyright © 2016 The Guilford Press. Reprinted by permission.

Over eight sessions, the therapist helped members to share their loving memories of Miguel as well as their grief at his tragic death. The sessions repaired the family's fragmentation, increasing the parents' mutual support and promoting more collaborative family teamwork in facing their bereavement challenges. The therapist also linked the parents with social services, which supported their efforts to obtain legal counsel and navigate the court system in their concerted actions to seek justice for the murder.

In the therapist's brief follow-up contact 6 months later, Teresa was doing well in school, and the father's drinking had abated. The experience of pulling together to deal with their loss had strengthened family bonds and was helping members to cope better with other stresses in their lives. A family check-in, held 6–12 months after a loss, can also be helpful in normalizing persisting grief and addressing common concerns, with unexpected arousal of intense emotions around a birthday, holiday, or anniversary of the death. The parents shared one worry: they dreaded Miguel's upcoming birthday. They were encouraged to gather with their extended family to remember him. The parents prepared his favorite foods and reminisced with aunts and uncles as the cousins sang and danced to Miguel's favorite music.

In communities affected by poverty, racism, and other forms of discrimination, violent deaths take a tragic toll, including wrongful deaths by police, especially with the senseless loss of young lives of promise (see Chapter 11). As bereaved families grapple with their intense sadness, clinicians need to be attentive to systemic roots and reverberations in their anger, frustration, and despair at racial injustice and inequities.

Increasingly, practitioners, beyond their work with individual families, are engaged in advocacy for needed changes in larger systems and for ending the epidemic of gun violence (Harris & Bordere, 2016).

Deaths Associated with Gender-Based and Domestic Violence

All too frequently, murders are committed by relatives or close acquaintances, mostly with firearms and often over personal grievances or suspected infidelities. High rates of murders are associated with gender-based violence, particularly for women and girls of color and highest for Indigenous women. Death resulting from serious abuse by a loved one is particularly devastating because it was inflicted by someone trusted and depended upon. Deaths in the context of relational abuse are predominantly the deaths of women by their male partners (NIA Project, Emory University, *https://psychiatry.emory.edu/niaproject*). Intimate partner violence affecting LGBTQI+ persons is grossly underreported due to a lack of awareness, stigma, and denial. Gender-based myths also perpetuate disbelief, such as assuming there aren't abusive lesbian relationships because women don't abuse each other.

The exact number of deaths in domestic violence incidents is uncertain due to denial of threats, failure to report them, or recanting by the abused person under pressure by their partner, who often vows to kill them if they follow through. When charges are brought, nearly 80% recant or change their testimony before the case reaches trial. The accuser is commonly released on bail, increasing risk to the partner, who often drops charges. In the complex cycles of violence and reconciliation in many relationships, each time the perpetrator promises to change but escalates patterns of intimidation, isolation, and abuse. Experts view choking as a predictor of mounting danger of death. Many factors influence a decision to leave, such as child welfare or financial dependency. Threats to kill a beloved pet if the abused partner leaves may keep the abused person in the relationship when shelters or alternate accommodations do not accept pets (see Chapter 8).

Of concern, the risk of death is heightened when the abused partner attempts to separate. Domestic violence–related homicides rise in the first year of separation and if/when the survivor starts another intimate relationship. Arrests and prosecutions are insufficient to lower the risk; orders for protection are too often violated, and consequently the accused lashes out, heightening the lethal risk.

Individual counseling is vitally important, as are access to shelters and relocation to ensure safety and attention to the protection of children and pets. Meetings that include trusted friends or extended family members may be helpful in preventing recurrence of cycles and risk. Most families, pained by the harm and recurrent threat, support attempts to leave abusive relationships. Yet, many become emotionally worn down by repeated cycles and legal hurdles. Some may encourage staying in the relationship, accepting minimizing accounts and the abuser's vows to change. Others are influenced by cultural or religious admonitions that a woman must be submissive to her husband's authority and must keep the family intact for the children. Family grief following a death may be complicated by self-recriminations for not doing more to protect them.

Drug-Related Deaths

Over the past decade, drug overdose deaths have increased threefold in the United States. In low-income and underresourced communities, predominantly people of color, multiple traumatic deaths of family members and friends, a bleak future outlook, and peer drug cultures all contribute to addiction. Lack of access to substance use treatment contributes to a rising rate of overdose deaths.

The opioid epidemic has become the leading cause of death for adults under age 55, taking more American lives than World Wars I and II combined. Research by leading economists (Case & Deaton, 2021) has found rising mortality rates for working-class Americans without a college degree. Called "deaths of despair," most deaths have been due to drug overdose, alcohol use, and suicide. The drug crisis, fueled by overprescribing pain medication, is intertwined with social ills, declines in job and economic prospects, and deteriorating physical and mental health.

Individuals who become addicted to prescription opioids often shift to heroin; drugs are increasingly laced with fentanyl, a deadly synthetic drug 50 times more potent than heroin. Synthetics added to other drugs, like cocaine, Xanax, and MDMA, have widened the epidemic and risk of overdose death in young people. Drugs have become easier to access online, attracting youth who are curious, and it has become more difficult for users to know what they are taking. As one mother related, "Our son was a wonderful kid who made a tragic mistake and got addicted. He tried to stop, and we tried to help him. Did he give up on life, or did he want to keep living? We'll never know."

Over time, addiction takes a toll on the family (Harrison & Connery, 2019). Complicated loss is common when a loved one has gone through treatments, relapses, and changes in personality, some with repeated deceptions or theft to support a habit. It can be an agonizing dilemma: how to support their loved one but not their addiction, whether to take them in (again) when they are homeless. Ambiguous losses are suffered over time—grieving the person and their relationships before addiction took hold—and with exhaustion and guilt-tinged relief when their death occurs.

When family members become blocked from healing by anger and despair after an overdose death, therapists can validate the complexity of their emotions and help them to reconnect with their loving concern for the deceased and find ways to honor them.

> Following his son's death from a drug overdose, Bert was consumed by rage and helplessness, not wanting to go on living. He had not been to his son's grave in the 2 years since the funeral because it was too painful. At his therapist's urging, he visited the grave, where he prayed for inspiration to guide his path ahead. That night he slept deeply for the first time since the death, dreamed of his son's joyful nature, and awoke with an awareness that his son would be ashamed of him, wasting away; he'd want him to do something worthwhile in his memory. With his therapist's encouragement, he turned self-destructive feelings into concerted action with other families and local authorities with the aim of stopping drug trafficking in their community.

Grieving Deaths by Suicide

Suicides can be tormenting for survivors, with the motives and suffering of the deceased often incomprehensible. Explanations for suicide seem insufficient. Loved ones left behind too often suffer unending guilt, spending years, and even a lifetime, imagining the final moments of life, guessing at motives, and berating themselves for the things they could (or should) have done that might have made a difference.

In the United States, suicide is the twelfth leading cause of death. Over the past decade, the suicide rate increased 33% (*www.nimh.nih.gov/health/statistics/suicide*). Suicide is widely underreported or is classified as accidental. For every completed suicide, many more people attempt suicide, often several times. Worldwide, women have higher rates of suicidal ideation and attempts, but men have higher rates of completed suicides, more often using firearms. Men are also less likely to seek help and are often not socialized to talk about their emotions.

Research finds a strong link between suicide and mood disorders and alcohol use disorders, with 25–50% of people with bipolar disorder attempting to end their lives. Yet, predicting who will die by suicide has eluded mental health researchers and practitioners. Notably, a prior suicide attempt is the highest risk factor for a completed suicide, particularly for those with intractable and unbearable emotional pain; yet most individuals who attempt suicide do not attempt again. Many suicides happen impulsively in moments of crisis with a breakdown in the ability to deal with life stresses, such as financial pressures, relationship breakup, or chronic pain and despair. Suicides may also be precipitated by unrecognized or unaddressed traumatic losses—the death of a loved one, the loss of a home, a livelihood, or financial solvency, and the lack of family and social support. Increasing disparities in income and healthcare are crucial factors in the feelings of despair, failure, and isolation that contribute to suicides.

Worldwide, experiences of conflict, disaster, violence, abuse, and traumatic loss are strongly associated with suicidal behavior. Suicide rates are high among vulnerable groups in humanitarian settings and among those who experience discrimination, such as racial minorities, refugees and migrants, and Indigenous peoples. In the United States, Native Americans have the highest rate of suicide. LGBTQI+ persons are at greater risk of suicide due to homophobia, transphobia, harassment, discrimination, and violence.

Suicide in Childhood and Adolescence

Over the past decade, suicide attempts among adolescents and younger children have been rising. Suicide is now the second leading cause of death in the United States for youth ages 15–19 years. With developing brains not yet equipping them to think long term or to look forward to better times, their immediate emotional pain can feel overwhelming and endless. Tending to act impulsively, they may act to end their distress.

Adverse experiences in childhood, such as physical, sexual, emotional abuse and neglect, violence, and family contexts impacted by mental health and substance abuse problems, are associated with an increased risk for suicide and suicide attempts in adolescence. Clinicians should pay attention to painful losses and dislocations with divorce, separation, or death of parents/guardians; frequent moves to a different residential area, school, and peer groups; and a family history of suicide. A high and persistent suicide risk is also associated with a lack of positive family and interpersonal relations and situations of peer bullying, peer-group pressure, and peer suicide, especially for gender-nonconforming teens. In all these situations, it's essential to address concerns and strengthen family support for youth who are at risk.

For gender-nonconforming or questioning youth, who often face peer bullying, their family's acceptance of their gender identity, questioning, and differences from social norms has been found to significantly reduce risks of suicide (Haas et al., 2010).

One mother sought therapy for herself after her transgender teenager, Dana, died by suicide. Her grief was unbearable, complicated by her husband's withdrawal and heavy drinking. She had lovingly accepted her child's identity, yet worried about the peer bullying they suffered. But her husband, unable to accept his son's change, harshly rejected Dana and refused further contact, which crushed Dana's spirit. The mother believed he blamed himself for Dana's death. The therapist encouraged her to invite him to meet together to share their complex grief and support each other.

Mental health emergencies and suicide attempts surged during the pandemic, particularly for those struggling with bullying, abuse, eating disorders, racism, or violence in their community. Social media also pose an increasing risk for youth, supporting ideas to hurt themselves or to end their lives. Algorithms connect them with other posts of sad kids, ways to self-harm, and suicide sites that suggest plans and methods. Girls, who are more likely to attempt suicide with an overdose of pills, are increasingly dying by firearms, as is the case for most boys. Therapists need to recognize that youths showing behavior problems may be covering depressed or suicidal feelings and need sensitive help the most. It's crucial to overcome barriers to prevention in the shortage of mental health professionals, inpatient and outpatient treatment, and affordable, community-based services.

Family involvement in therapy is crucial for preventing suicide for youth experiencing suicidal thoughts and behaviors. Family connectedness, emotional support, and monitoring reduce risk. Individual treatment can include a family component or multifamily groups. Family sessions aim to reduce negative family and social influences and to strengthen family functioning and cohesive, supportive relationships, fostering a sense of belonging, mutual caring, and commitment. Families can be crucial therapeutic allies in building youth skills in coping, problem solving, and conflict management, as well as encouraging positive social connections with peers, teachers, and mentoring adults to counter oppressive conditions and encourage steps toward positive future aims (Walsh, 2016c).

Suicide in College-Age Young Adults

Suicide is also the second leading cause of death (after accidents) among college-age young adults in the United States. The number of students seeking treatment for anxiety and depression has risen sharply over the past few years. The ripple effects of suicide for peers in academic settings also require attention and outreach.

Drew was found dead in his dorm room, where he had been studying for final exams and was anxious about his grades. His death sent shock waves through the student community, identifying with the pressures he was under. A common reaction was, "It could have been me." Rumors circulated that his death was drug related. School officials released minimal information to the university community in a misguided attempt to allay concerns of risk by other students, their families, and alumni. The cause of death—whether medical, accidental or intentional—was not announced, leaving ambiguity that complicated their meaning-making and mourning processes. At the end of the term, a student in his study group sent an email response to the expressions of sympathy and support they had received from one professor:

> Thank you for caring. The tragic death of our friend and classmate has been very difficult—yet coming together in our loss has been rich and healing, as well. The first several weeks felt hazy. The shock is gradually wearing off, leading to a deeper sense of sadness but acceptance, too. I often feel like I see him around campus. He's still very much in our thoughts. I've woven a stone he gave me from his summer trip on the bracelet I wear, so that I can keep him in mind. He was a rare character—funny, whimsical, sensitive, creative, and brilliant. There also seemed a deep sadness, although rarely revealed, and I don't think we understand the private struggles he endured. We organized a service, which was very powerful and so appropriate to capture his spirit—it really helped the whole student body and faculty. My cohort, which has always been close, has pulled together even more, and we hope to do something positive with what has happened, in his name.

Drew's parents' grief was heavy with incomprehension; it made no sense to them—he was always smiling and cheerful and a top student with a promising future. A month later, his mother found her son's journal in the box of belongings returned to them. As the first in his family to go to college, he wrote about the constant pressure to excel through high school and college, to be a "star." He was flunking three courses as he struggled to sleep, missed classes, and turned in assignments late. He felt like a total failure. He hid his self-doubts and spiraling depression, expecting his family's crushing disappointment in him. One instructor, noticing his distress, suggested he get counseling, but he was on a long waiting list in the understaffed student clinic. His mother's discovery set off waves of pain and soul-searching. It also propelled the parents to campaign for more proactive and accessible student mental health services and revisions to college policies of confidentiality intended to protect students' privacy (and the college's reputation) for more forthright communications with their families and the concerned student and faculty community.

While respecting privacy concerns, it is important that educational and work systems not cover up a stigmatized cause of death, particularly if the death is drug-related or a possible suicide. Fears and fantasies of the worst tend to circulate through informal networks. It's vital to respond to the grief and concerns in families and the relational network of students and faculty and to facilitate community memorial events. Open acknowledgment and discussion of the situation foster healing and facilitate institutional changes to reduce risks and prevent future tragedies.

Suicide in Adulthood and Later Life

The conviction that suffering is irremediable is common among adults who are suicidal. Some act to end their life to free themselves from unendurable pain. Often, they hide their suffering behind a veil of cheer, flashing a big smile; yet they may reveal a shadow of suffering. Many varied factors may contribute, such as career or financial downturns that fuel depression, hopelessness, loss of meaning, guilt, or shame. At high risk are those who think they've made a mess of everything and are powerless to fix it. Men living alone and recently divorced or widowed are at higher risk. In persons with an underlying mood disorder, the risk is worsened by alcohol or substance use. Some who have tried psychotherapy, psychotropic medications, and psychiatric treatments, such as electroconvulsive therapy, feel that nothing has helped. Of note, persons psychiatrically hospitalized for depression and suicidal ideation are at high risk of suicide shortly after discharge.

Some think that their loved ones would be better off without them and those in addictions treatment may even be advised that they shouldn't change for others, only for themselves. It's crucial for clinicians to expand consideration to the devastating impact their suicide would likely have for a loving parent, a spouse, or especially their children.

One client, Brandon, was angry, despondent, and suicidal, after his wife left him and moved away with their children, whom he had not seen for several months. He acknowledged some wish to hurt his "ex" by causing her guilt for the divorce and his death. I engaged him in conversations about his children, from memories of their early childhood to their recent teens, focusing on his love for them and theirs for him. He wept openly, sharing how much he missed them, saying it was too upsetting to hear their voices, for him to call them often. I asked how losing contact from him might be for them. He imagined how devastating it would be—they might think he didn't care about them or even feel abandoned by him. We then considered the impact for them if they lost him forever to suicide, realizing they would never see him again, and might even blame themselves. Contemplating the long-term pain and suffering he would cause them, he firmly vowed that he would not end his life—he could never do that to them. I suggested that he post their photos on his refrigerator to inspire him every day in his efforts to move forward in his life. He also began calling them weekly, and they started regular internet exchanges, sharing brief messages, cartoons, and photos, with plans to visit in the coming months.

In some cases, chronic, debilitating medical conditions, entailing multiple losses, may lead to despair.

Mick, a construction worker left permanently disabled by a workplace accident, was drinking heavily. One night, his wife, Peg, found him passed out on the floor, with his hunting rifle ready to be fired. In individual and conjoint sessions, we explored the multiple losses he had experienced: the sense of productivity and camaraderie with coworkers on his job, his family role as breadwinner, and his sexual functioning and active leisure life.

  In family sessions, his wife and children helped him realize how much he was loved, valued, and needed, which was crucial to his healing and resilience. Their support recharged his will to live and reorient his life to make the most of his possibilities. With his family's encouragement, Mick found new ways to be productive and active. As Peg increased her job from part-time to full-time status, he took on more active coparenting and household coordination, finding new satisfactions in cooking and in closer bonds. Over time, he set up a web-based small business and began coaching his daughter's soccer team. He told Peg that although he never would have wished for his disability, his life and loved ones now meant more to him than ever before.

The suicide rate among U.S. military service members and veterans, most often by lethal weapons, has risen alarmingly over the past decade. While varied personal influences may be involved, more often suicides are associated with debilitating medical injuries and psychological wounds, as in PTSD. The highest incidence is among those suffering *moral injury*—an anguished sense of unworthiness in conduct that violates deeply held moral values, especially in the killing of women and children (Griffin et al., 2019; see Chapter 11).

  Suicide rates are also high among older adult men and women, especially those over age 75, widowed, and alone. Limited social contact is associated with suicidal ideation, underscoring the importance of mobilizing ongoing kin and social connections, both in person and through cards and letters, calls, and the internet. Chronic, painful, and debilitating health conditions, unaffordable medical treatments and medications, and concerns of overburdening family members may also be contributing factors. Clinicians need to listen well to concerns that may lead someone to want to end their life.

Overcoming Social Stigma; Addressing the Family Impact

The social stigma surrounding mental disorders and suicide keeps many people from seeking help when they are thinking of taking their own life or after they have made an attempt. Many are reluctant to openly discuss it, particularly if details seem unsavory or deaths are judged unworthy or unjustified. Raising community awareness and breaking down barriers are important. In referring to suicide, phrases such as "attempted suicide," "died by suicide," and "took their own life" are advised rather than "*commit* suicide," which increases stigma, suggests criminal actions, and discourages people from seeking help. Also, it is advisable not to label as "suicide" a person's wishes for assisted dying measures near the end of life for dignity and control in the dying process (see Chapter 4).

Bereaved families experience more stigma and less social support after a suicide than after all other types of loss. Too often they experience further trauma by police interrogations and media attention at the scene of the death and in the immediate aftermath, when they are overwhelmed and in a state of shock and extreme distress. They are likely to face public exposure of those most private moments and their immediate reactions, as happened to the actress Ashley Judd and her family:

> My beloved mother, Naomi Judd, who had come to believe that her mental illness would only get worse, never better, took her own life that day. The trauma of discovering and then holding her laboring body haunts my nights. As my family and I continue to mourn our loss, the rampant and cruel misinformation that has spread about her death, and about our relationships with her, stalks my days. (Judd, 2022)

Social interactions can be awkward and avoided, with spoken or implied judgment, cruel insinuations, and blame: "Well, maybe if you hadn't . . . " Concerns about religious condemnation of suicide may also contribute to coverup (see Chapter 10). Concealing the cause of death can distort family communication, strain their relations, and leave members struggling on their own to deal with the experience. Clinicians can be helpful in addressing these concerns and repairing estranged bonds (see Chapter 10).

For families, the loss of a loved one to suicide is tormenting when it appears impulsive, senseless, or intended to hurt others (Jordan & McIntosh, 2011; Kaslow, Samples, Rhodes, & Gantt, 2011). There is a heightened search for meaning in their struggle to understand why and to make sense of the death. Commonly, family members grapple with feelings of responsibility and blame, ruminating over how they might have made a difference. When there was conflict with the deceased, guilt and regret may predominate. For some, feelings of abandonment or unlovability may surface. A child may question, "If my dad loved me enough, he wouldn't have left me like that."

For some families, a suicide is a unique event; if they never contemplated the possibility, the death shatters their core assumptions. They may flounder in a state of confusion as they grieve. In cases of serious mental illness or addiction, families may have been aware of the risk for some time and afraid that their loved one, who may have threatened to end their life, would actually do so. Commonly, when a loved one struggles over a long time, the bereaved feel guilt-tinged relief that their psychological pain is over, as well as the heartache and disruptions in the family. Family therapist David Treadway (2004, 2022) has written about this overwhelming complexity of feelings, based on his extensive work with families in the aftermath of suicide and informed by his own long struggle after his mother took her own life. Bonds can be splintered as each individual responds in their own way: "Some weep; some blame; some drink; some break. Some just shut down entirely. Like a power surge in the electrical system, the fuse blows and the lights go out" (Treadway, 2004, p. 398). Clinicians should be aware of an increased risk of self-destructive behavior, suicidal ideation, and attempts by loved ones most directly affected by a suicide. It's crucial to explore family histories of traumatic deaths that may heighten the risk of suicide for a spouse, parent, child, or sibling, particularly at an anniversary or birthday (see Chapter 7).

Therapists can be helpful by facilitating family members' understanding of the complex nature of suicide and the possible contribution of many intersecting factors. We can encourage members to share their experience and gradually accept that certain questions may never be answered. Some couples break apart in their unbearable grief with the traumatic death of a child. While individuals may have different perspectives or emotional reactions, helping them share their loss experience can repair strains and foster mutual understanding.

> Jeremy came for therapy after his 17-year-old son took his own life. The day after the funeral, his wife, Ellie, without consulting him, emptied out the son's room, disposing of all his clothing and belongings. It was too

painful for her to see any reminder of their son and his absence. Jeremy was in agony, bewildered by the death and furious with his wife. As their conflict escalated, Ellie insisted that he move out and take his belongings with him. Individual and joint sessions were combined to interrupt their escalation, reconsider disruptive moves, help each to express their own deep pain, and encourage their mutual support.

In my practice, I've seen the remarkable resilience forged from deep suffering through new purpose and activism to prevent a similar tragedy for others. In striving to make something good come out of their suffering, such efforts also enhance meaning, connection, and feelings of reempowerment, as in the following instance:

> One couple came for counseling, distraught after their talented and beloved 28-year-old daughter, suffering with bipolar disorder, took her life. Their pain, anger, and self-blame gradually eased as they gained understanding of her mental health challenges, with intolerable oscillation between manic highs and deep depression. At the first anniversary of her death, they contacted me, expressing the strong need to do something positive in her memory. They set up a foundation in her name for suicide prevention, mobilizing their faith congregation to hold an annual public event to increase awareness and decrease stigma around mental illness and suicide. They saw this as a way to honor their daughter's life and to channel their pain and sorrow to spare other families a similar tragedy. Their faith community continued to be a bedrock of support.

Socioeconomic, Cultural, and Religious Influences

Current mental health approaches focus largely on the individual, identifying persons at risk and referring them for mental healthcare. Interventions should address contextual factors, from complex relational dynamics to socioeconomic variables and racial oppression that may influence suicide risk and bereavement adaptation, such as job loss and financial strains, and access to healthcare and mental health services.

It is important for clinicians to explore cultural and religious influences in suicide risk and in stigma and attitudes toward help seeking with suicide (see Chapter 3). For Asian Americans, the loss of "face"—one's prestige and position in society—can prompt suicidal thoughts and actions related to shame that one has brought on the family name and standing. Such reasons for suicide are common among Asian men who have experienced loss of status in their careers and for adolescents who fail performance expectations on exams that determine their future prospects. The sense of shame also keeps at-risk individuals and their families from seeking help.

In immigrant families, the clash between old and new values commonly sparks intergenerational conflict (Falicov, 2014). In some traditional cultures, this can escalate to lethal threats, particularly for adolescent girls and women suspected of sexual impropriety. They may be expected to take their own life to restore the family honor (commonly by stabbing, hanging, or self-immolation) or face the threat of an honor killing by a male relative. Some run away, estranged from the family, vulnerable on their own, and at risk of sexual trafficking.

> I once consulted with a refugee mental health center staff in a European city, where a counselor presented concerns about a Kurdish family. The mother and her teenage son and daughter, who arrived a year earlier, had resettled successfully. Family conflict arose when the father recently joined them. He was furious with the daughter for socializing with male and female friends in cafes and public venues, as was typical for local teenagers but was forbidden in their traditional culture. The father–daughter conflict escalated, with the mother trying to make peace. In the past week, the daughter awoke one morning to find a knife on her bedside table. The counselor, unfamiliar with their culture and seeing the daughter's behavior as normal from his own cultural standpoint, was concerned about how to respond to the situation. I urged him to consider this threat seriously and to respond immediately to prevent a tragedy. In the consultation group, we discussed ways to respectfully explore and address cross-cultural differences in resettlement and across generations.

Confluence of Traumatic and Threatened Losses in Multistressed Families

Crisis situations in multistressed, low-income families often involve a confluence of challenging conditions, with the convergence of traumatic past losses and current threatened loss, as in the following case (Walsh, 2016b):

> Jamar, age 11, lived with his grandmother and her partner in a public housing complex. In recent months, his frequent school absences and failing grades worried his school staff that he was hanging out in the streets. As is common in low-income, marginalized communities, when there was no response to calls and notes sent home, the family was presumed likely to be dysfunctional and uncaring. A school social worker in our program, assigned to the case, made a home visit to assess the situation. Jamar and his brother and sister lived with their grandmother, their legal guardian since their mother's death in a drug overdose 4 years earlier. The grandmother had been hospitalized 3 months ago with a serious liver disease and kidney failure; now at home, she required dialysis

several times a week. Jamar, who had been very close to his mother, was cut off from his father since her death, and was now extremely anxious that he might also lose his grandmother. He was missing school to watch over her.

The worker also noted that the burden of responsibility for the children heightened risk for the grandmother's fragile health. No one talked about her precarious condition, the threat of another loss and dislocation for the children, or possible arrangements for their care in the event of her death. As Jamar said, "It was all just too scary."

Genogram construction (see Figure 9.2) was helpful to diagram this complex family situation and to identify potential resources. The worker took several steps to help the family with its crisis. Most immediate was the need to reduce the risk factors and shore up resources for the grandmother's health and the children's care. The grandmother's cohabiting partner had not been involved with them, but now, worried about her declining health, he agreed to take a more active role to relieve her burden. A maternal aunt, contacted to be part of a team effort, took Jamar after school to do homework with her son.

The children's father, blamed for the mother's drug-related death, had been cut off by the grandmother. With her assent, he was contacted to assess his current ability and desire to assume any parenting role. His deep remorse at his wife's death had spurred him to give up drug use and get his life in order. Now stable and employed, he yearned for contact with his children. The counselor facilitated his reconciliation with the family. With steps to restore trust and to monitor safety, he became actively involved with all three children, each at risk and responsive to his positive investment. As immediate stresses were reduced, all members were benefiting from the strengthened family network. Counseling addressed the children's anxieties about losing their grandmother, commingled with grief over their mother's death. Attention turned to their future hopes and concerns and possibilities for residence with their father.

This case illustrates how resilience-based interventions in a very complex situation can foster both individual and family well-being by addressing core elements in the three domains of family functioning: meaning making and mastery of the crisis; reorganization of family structural patterns; and more effective communication and problem solving.

ADDRESSING LARGER SYSTEMIC INFLUENCES

Our society views homicide, suicide, and alcohol- and drug-related deaths primarily in terms of bad individual choices, due to mental illness or personal failings. Risks are too readily presumed due to family dysfunction.

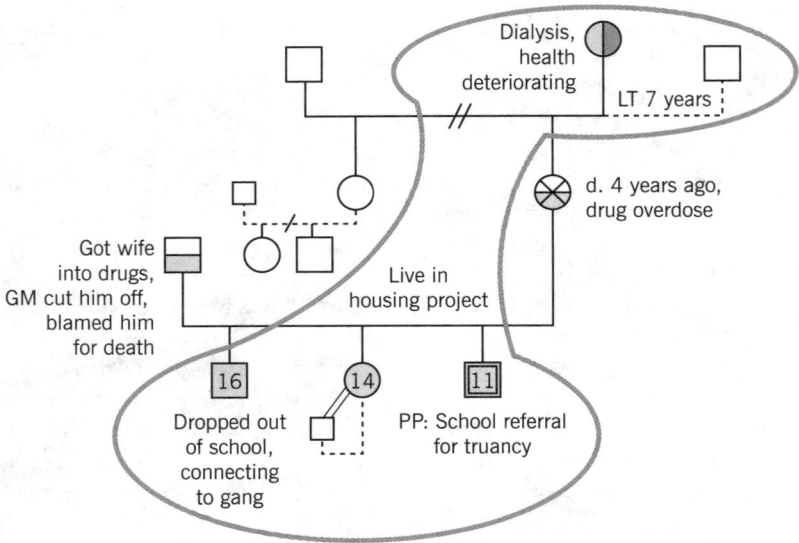

FIGURE 9.2. Genogram of the complex family situation of Jamar, referred to counseling for truancy. From Walsh (2016b). Copyright © 2016 The Guilford Press. Reprinted by permission.

As one mother sobbed, "I wish people could see our pain without condemning my son's actions or presuming our fault as bad parents. Our life is shattered." As clinicians, we need to gain understanding of our clients' lived experience in their social contexts. In many cases, social pressures and/or structural impediments, such as stigma, violence, vulnerability, discrimination, and exploitation, contribute to high death rates.

Greater attention is needed to pervasive structural factors linked to social and economic inequities. Among those who die in homicide and by suicide, there are stark and increasing racial disparities, particularly for youth. Greater attention is needed to the stress, trauma, anger, and despair experienced by Black, Indigenous, and other communities of color. An ever-present threat—of neighborhood violence, police shootings, microaggressions, and injustices—can enrage and wound the spirit (Hardy, 2023). Youth growing up in poor, marginalized, and blighted neighborhoods may become hopeless about their future. The high risk of early violent death, especially for young males, fuels doubts about even reaching adulthood.

The high rate of gun violence and deaths in the United States is fueled by the pervasive gun culture and the proliferation of firearms with easy access. Keeping weapons unloaded and locked greatly reduces accidental deaths, homicide, and suicide among gun owners and all family members. The urgent need for strict gun safety laws and restrictions on assault weapons requires concerted public attention and action to stop the epidemic of shootings in our streets, our schools, our places of worship, and our public spaces.

THE CRISIS OF MEANING AND CONNECTION IN TRAUMATIC LOSS: FOSTERING HEALING AND RESILIENCE

Situations of traumatic death pose high risk for complicated bereavement and require careful assessment and sensitive intervention, applying the practice principles offered in Chapters 2 and 5. What does it mean to encourage survivors to express and share their experience of profound loss? We attend to the varying emotions and implications for members and for the family unit. With respect for cultural, family, and personal differences, we can help them sort out in what ways and with whom to share their experience as they chart their path forward.

When traumatic loss is suffered, families may gain partial "closure" on some aspects, such as learning more about the circumstances of a death, but they rarely experience "resolution" or completely get over it. Healing and resilience involve complex, gradual, and fluid processes over time, with various facets of grief alternating and reemerging with unexpected intensity, particularly around significant events and anniversaries.

Our work with bereaved individuals, couples, and families aims not only to help them understand and reduce emotional, physical, or relational distress in the wake of loss, but also to assist them in reconstructing a coherent narrative for themselves and their world at psychological, social, cultural, and spiritual levels. As grief and healing processes progress, we can encourage their increasing focus on ways to affirm life and to reorient and adapt to include the loss but not be dominated by it. Reengagement in employment and activities that give a sense of structure and meaning enhances a positive sense of self and appreciation of life. As we've seen in many cases, the tragedy can spark new purpose. Therapists can listen for such sparks of inspiration: the urge to make a difference, to dedicate actions for something good to come out of a tragedy.

A challenge in meaning making is that violent and traumatic losses shatter basic core constructs or our "assumptive world" on which we rely (Janoff–Bulman, 1992). Our taken-for-granted sense of security, predictability, and trust are profoundly disrupted by the experience. The invalidation of abiding beliefs strips away illusory assumptions that once sustained us and also poses profound challenges to our sense of identity and self-continuity over time. A senseless tragedy is especially hard to bear.

Coming to terms with the loss does not necessarily mean that survivors must make sense of that loss. It can reflect a new wisdom from experience and a testament to strengths that have been forged. In our work, we may need to help people envision a new sense of normality, identity, and relatedness to adapt to altered conditions. Our task is not to make meaning for them, but to support their efforts to find their own meaning out of their experience.

A systemic approach to loss considers the biopsychosocial effects of violent, life-ending events, the varying experience for loved ones, and the impact on the family unit and relational networks. Therapeutic efforts aim to facilitate grieving processes, to reorient hope from a bleak outlook, and to find meaning and energy to reengage in relationships and life pursuits. Although therapists and loved ones cannot always prevent a violent death, the risks can be lessened by opening communication and mobilizing relational support. Therapeutic efforts aim to strengthen couple and family adaptation and tap community, cultural, and spiritual resources for healing and resilience.

In so many cases, a tragedy can open new horizons, as families channel their grief into new purpose to honor the memory of their loved one by advocating for research, treatment, and prevention to benefit others. Therapists can listen for such inspiration: the urge to make a difference, to act so that something good can come out of a tragedy and, in doing so, further a family's own healing and resilience.

CHAPTER 10

Addressing Complex Relational and Transgenerational Dynamics

Reverberations from the Past

> Never. We never lose our loved ones. They accompany us; they don't disappear from our lives. We are merely in different rooms.
>
> —PAULO COELHO, *Aleph*

Like the social context, the temporal context holds a matrix of meanings in which all behavior is embedded. As we've seen, a significant loss can fuel strong reactions affecting survivors' life pursuits and other relationships. In my experience, it's not helpful to refer to such bereavement complications as "unresolved mourning," since complete resolution is rarely attained and it sets up unrealistic expectations for therapy and for life going forward.

Many factors can contribute to long-term effects with a deeply troubling loss experience. Beyond immediate grief reactions, emotional shock waves can reverberate throughout relational networks long after a death, even across generations. Attention to this underground shock wave is important in therapy when people seek help long after a significant death, often presenting other concerns (Walsh & McGoldrick, 2004). It is more likely to be problematic when the past loss and grief had not been handled well in the family. In other cases, a more recent or threatened death and loss may reactivate long-dormant family dynamics related to earlier losses or traumatic experiences.

LONG-TERM IMPACT OF FAMILY MALADAPTIVE
RESPONSE TO TRAUMATIC LOSS

How a family responds to loss and facilitates emotional sharing, meaning-making, reorganization, and reinvestment in life forward will influence the long-term adaptation for members and their relationships. A family's maladaptive response (see Chapter 5) can shut down communication and support for members' grief and undermine their meaning making, with painful reverberations. This impact for children after the traumatic death of a parent is seen in the following interviews (Senior, 2020), nearly two decades after the death by suicide of a prominent psychologist:

> Philip Brickman, an academic expert on the pursuit of happiness, had a productive career and seemingly idyllic family life, yet he suffered periods of depression. In midcareer, with the loss of a grant and the loss of his marriage, he was despondent and isolated, living in a grim apartment. He told colleagues he thought of killing himself—but then joked about it, disarming their concern. He sought inpatient psychiatric treatment, but after signing himself out, he jumped to his death from the tallest building in town—across from his office. (That day, he was scheduled to meet with his estranged wife for a couple therapy session.)
>
> In interviews 18 years later with his daughters, they recalled that upon their father's death, their mother never again spoke of him, discussed his death, or visited his grave. They regretted most that she had not guided them in grieving or helped them know or love their father. She later changed her name, moved away, became a nurse, and told others that her husband had died of cancer.
>
> One daughter, closest to the father, had sensed his sorrow as a little girl and tried to help, in her own way, by letting him win at cards. She carried into adulthood a common misunderstanding by children: that her father's suicide was her fault, that she should have been able to save him. When she reached 30, she realized that he wanted to leave, and it was his right. "It wasn't about me."
>
> Another daughter reflected that she kept finding men who were somehow broken and needed saving. Her few memories of her father were painful, as when he begged her to ask her mother whether she still loved him. She recalled sitting in his office and asking what would happen if she fell out of one of the big windows. She couldn't remember his response, but soon after, he jumped from the tower. Asked if she believed she might have seeded a family tragedy, she first said no, not really. She knew her father had tried suicide before. "But if I did, what a jerk!" she blurted out. "Did he think that wouldn't negatively affect me for the rest of my life?" It was the first time that she'd said this thought out loud.

Still, she remained mostly protective of her father and angry with her mother for not helping them to grieve.

Brickman's sister was also deeply affected by the silence surrounding the death. It took her a decade to stop imagining his jump. Asked how she coped with the common self-questioning of survivors for things done or not done, she said it took years of therapy to feel reassured that she had not done anything terrible. It consoled her that when she last saw him, she treated him with love, support, and kindness.

In traumatic deaths (see Chapter 9), bereaved loved ones often seek help many years later with death-related issues still unclear and painful. Therapists can be helpful in facilitating meaning making, mutual support, and both individual and relational healing.

In one family I worked with, Emily, age 33, called to request family sessions for herself and her siblings with their father, Walter. Since they left home for college, they had all been estranged, with only superficial conversation at holiday visits. They wanted to know the truth about their mother's death when they were in their early teens. Their father had told them that she had died peacefully in her sleep during the night when her heart gave out. In his grief, he didn't want to talk about it further, and communication shut down in family life, with increasing emotional distance, leaving each to deal with the loss on their own. They never understood what had happened and had overheard relatives' whispered suspicions of suicide, with an overdose of prescription drugs. The ambiguity gnawed away at Emily over time, as she imagined different possible scenarios and couldn't make sense of why her mother would have ended her life. The father's recent heart attack prompted them to act now, fearing that after his death they would never know the truth.

Walter was open to a meeting, as he longed for more connection with his adult children and barely knew his grandchildren. For the first time, Emily directly asked the question no one had dared to pose: "Did Mom take her own life?" He hesitated, with discomfort, but then told them the truth. Their mother had suffered from severe bouts of depression. She had tried to end her life once before, when he had been able to stop her. But this time she hid the bottle of prescription pills taken at bedtime and died in her sleep. She had loved them all very much, but her pain was too great for her to bear. Still, he blamed himself for failing to make her happy enough to keep living, and he still carried that anguish.

Walter told them he covered up the suicide because he didn't want to upset the children further after losing their mother. And the social stigma would have been rough for them to face. Worst of all were his religious concerns: if the death had been declared a suicide, their mother, as a Catholic, couldn't have received last rites or be buried in the cemetery with their family. So, he decided it was best, for her sake as well, to hide the truth. Over time, carrying his guilty secret, he distanced from his pastor and left his congregation. He now felt alone in the world.

With deep sincerity, Walter apologized to his children for withholding the truth from them. As time passed, he had wanted to tell them, but with so little contact, it never seemed to be a good time to bring up the painful past. The siblings, at first upset that he had lied, realized that in their devastating loss, his intentions were to do what he believed would be easier for them to bear and protect them from hurtful repercussions. The family sessions brought them all to deeper understanding and closer bonds.

I also encouraged Walter to meet with his former pastor, to share openheartedly the whole truth. He was deeply relieved by the pastor's compassion for the complicated situation and his plight, welcoming him back into his faith community. Church strictures around suicide had changed, and the pastor urged him to share his experience with other parishioners to decrease stigma and foster greater openness, understanding, and support of others at risk and their families.

INFLUENCE OF PAST LOSS
IN CURRENT PRESENTING PROBLEMS

In our early research and clinical experience over several decades, Monica McGoldrick and I both found that a traumatic past loss can be a significant influence in other problems that bring people to therapy years later (Walsh, 1983; McGoldrick & Walsh, 1983; Walsh & McGoldrick, 1988, 2004, 2013). Clients presenting current individual issues, relational distress, or child-focused problems may not mention the past loss experience, often unaware of its possible connection. A clinician's narrow focus on the current crisis and observable here-and-now relational patterns can blind notice of the potential relevance of a critical past loss and surrounding family dynamics.

With a systemic perspective, it's important for clinicians to understand the relational and temporal contexts of presenting problems. When clients present concerns around separation, attachment, or commitment, it is particularly important to explore possible connections to earlier traumatic losses. The death of a previous spouse can evoke catastrophic fears of loss in a later marriage, as in the following case:

Vic, widowed when his first wife died after the spread of metastatic breast cancer, remarried happily to Mallory. Unfortunately, a year later, Mallory was diagnosed with early-stage breast cancer. Vic immediately took flight from the relationship, unable to be intimate or support her emotionally. He then moved out, leaving a note saying that he just could not go through it all again and couldn't bear another loss. Although their marriage did not survive, Mallory's cancer did not recur, and she went on to thrive in her life. Vic, living alone, avoided other intimate attachments and eventually sought therapy for loneliness and depression.

In other cases, the ending of a current relationship arouses intense emotions from an earlier unmourned loss, leading a person to seek therapy. Samantha, age 28, had barely grieved her mother's death 5 years earlier, consumed by heavy job demands, and she married soon after. Now, at the breakup of her marriage, she experienced an unexpected flood of submerged emotions over her mother's death. It's important for therapists to attend to both losses and the intertwined grief.

In some cases, earlier family dynamics around a tragic loss contribute to later difficulties in life strivings, as in the following case:

Brian, age 33, sought therapy for a repeated cycle of setting grandiose career goals that he pursued at a fevered pitch, only to undermine himself each time he was on the brink of success. He didn't know why this kept happening. In exploring his family relations, he said he still felt extreme discomfort whenever he went home to visit his parents. The family room was like a "shrine" to his older brother, who had been killed in military combat at age 21. Pictures, medals, and plaques covered the walls. Brian felt a strong (unspoken) expectation to fulfill his parents' dreams for their firstborn son—yet he sensed a counter injunction that it would be disloyal to achieve in life what his brother was denied. Individual therapy focused on shifting his triangulated position, helping him and his parents to unknot his bind.

In approaching family history, a systemic perspective requires an evolutionary view, considering multiple, mutually interacting influences over time and in social context. Therapists need to be mindful not to assume a deterministic causal effect, that is, that current difficulties are due to a past adverse loss experience. It's crucial not to reduce understanding of complex situations to any single cause–effect. We don't interpret client experience or provide meaning; we notice and inquire about critical events and relational patterns to explore their potential meaning and significance for them.

Life-Cycle Convergence with Past Death/Loss Experience

Distress is heightened when a current milestone in life passage reactivates painful memories and emotions from an earlier death at the same point in the family life cycle. Individuals may lose perspective and conflate immediate situations with past events, sometimes out of awareness. Sketching a family genogram and timeline with clients (see Chapter 5) can facilitate exploration of significant past events and their relevance to current distress. Noting the dates of birth and death of important family members can prompt inquiry about a painful past loss.

Individuals commonly become anxious about their own (or their spouse's) threatened mortality upon reaching the same age or life transition at which a parent died. Many start new fitness regimens or make abrupt career or relationship changes. Some show sudden interest in high-risk adventures, such as sky diving, to deny—or take control—of the threat looming barely out of awareness, linked to a past loss. Catastrophic fears are common. One man, whose father, had died at 47, lived fearful of early death until he turned 48, feeling enormous relief thereafter. One couple, in their 60s, came for therapy in intense conflict over the husband's keen wish to retire and his wife's adamant opposition. In taking a brief family history, we noted that her father had died just after his retirement. As she realized her concern about losing her husband, it was important to consider the husband's health risks and differentiate the two situations in coming to a shared decision.

Reverberations of Past Sibling Loss in a Life-Threatening Crisis

Clinicians should note family histories of traumatic losses that may heighten the risk of suicide, particularly at an anniversary, birthday, or significant milestone. Often, past losses are not mentioned in presenting problems or initial assessment.

> Jeff, age 14, was hospitalized after an overdose, by taking a handful of his mother's pain pills. He and his parents were at a loss to understand why he did it. In a meeting with the parents, when asked to describe their family, they noted Jeff and his younger sister, but made no mention of an older son. In an individual session with Jeff, he began talking about his brother Peter, who had died in a car crash at age 14. In a family session, when asked about Peter, the parents were hazy around the date or events of the death, saying they had tried to put it out of their minds. Jeff then described how he had tried to take his brother's place to ease his parents' loss. They never spoke of Peter, but he could see the sorrow in their eyes. He wore his brother's handed-down clothes and cultivated his appearance to resemble old photos he kept in a drawer. When he turned 14, the age at which his brother had died, he said he was changing from the way he was "supposed to look," and he didn't know "how to be" anymore. Despairing and confused, he could only think to join his brother in heaven. Therapy, combining separate and joint sessions,

focused on enabling Jeff and his parents to deal with the past loss and relinquish his surrogate position so that he could move forward in his own development.

The Role of the Extended Family in Bereavement Complications

It's important to view the family network as an evolving system, moving forward in time. With a devastating loss, relational dynamics involving the extended family can complicate bereavement and prolong grief, sometimes for years, with later symptoms bringing a family to therapy (see Figure 10.1).

> Mrs. Lowe brought her 4-year-old son, Danny, to the child clinic because he refused to start preschool and had uncontrollable tantrums each morning. In taking a family history, the therapist learned that an older brother, Devon, had died at the same age, 3 years earlier, after developing a high fever from a virus he had contracted in preschool. The paternal grandparents, in their grief, blamed her for not having been sufficiently attentive to their adored first grandson, despite the pediatrician's assurance that she had not been at fault. Her in-laws refused to have her in their home, with continuing hostility. Mr. Lowe, torn between loyalty to his parents and his wife, distanced from her. Isolated in her grief, she continued to celebrate Devon's birthdays with Danny,

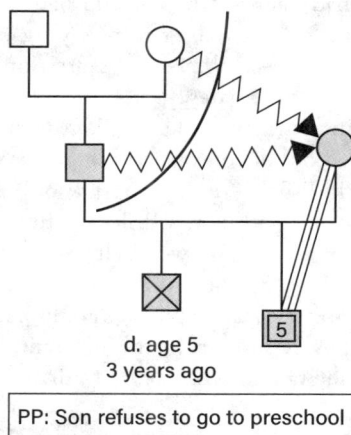

d. age 5
3 years ago

PP: Son refuses to go to preschool

FIGURE 10.1. Genogram showing extended family dynamics in presenting problems (PP) and connection to past loss. From Walsh (2016c). Copyright © 2016 The Guilford Press. Reprinted by permission.

each year making a birthday cake with candles for the age Devon would have been. Her silent self-recriminations fueled anxious overprotection of Danny when he was to start preschool.

Therapists should carefully evaluate the meaning of presenting problems to explore past life experiences that may be interconnected. A family genogram and timeline can be useful to visualize and address complex relational patterns.

Transgenerational Reactivation of Past Traumatic Loss

When ambiguous circumstances of a past traumatic death contribute to later distress, therapists can coach clients on seeking out more information, bringing greater clarity and peace of mind. In the following case, concerns surfaced when the client's daughter reached the same age as his sister had been at her traumatic death:

> Dennis, in his early 40s, was having recurrent nightmares over recent months about the death of his sister Roseanne, at age 17, in a car crash. He now worried constantly about the safety of his teenage daughter, Rose—named for his sister—and imagined every sort of traffic accident. The circumstances of his sister's death were ambiguous; his parents had arranged a closed-casket funeral, and no one in his family had wanted to talk about it. In our work together, I encouraged Dennis to locate his sister's friend who had been in the car and had survived the accident. At first, he was doubtful of finding him, saying it was "like a needle in a haystack." Urged to ask others and search online, he reached the friend's mother, who immediately put him in touch with the friend. He was open and informative: Their buddy driving the car had been drinking and swerved out of control, crashing into a tree. Roseanne had died instantly of a skull fracture. The friend, only slightly injured, had tended to her and stayed with her. While painful to hear how she died, Dennis had always imagined the worst. It brought him peace of mind to learn more about the accident and the care shown to his sister. It also reduced his global anxiety that "anything could happen at any time" to his daughter. Drawing lessons from the incident, he drove more cautiously himself, and he taught Rose never to drink and drive.

It's crucial for therapists to explore the potential significance of past loss events that are unmentioned in clients' presenting problems. In some cases, a client may be reluctant to revisit a traumatic past loss or may initially insist that it has no relevance. An active therapeutic approach is needed, with sensitivity to client priorities and hesitations.

Steve, age 38, was married, with an 8-year-old son. He came to therapy to stop his recent heavy drinking and an extramarital affair because, he said, he feared he was on the verge of losing everything important to him. As we explored this, he said, "Well my wife would leave me and I couldn't bear to lose my son, Mikey. He's the joy of my life."

In sketching a family genogram, I noted that Steve's younger brother, named Michael, had died at age 8. I wondered if there might be any connection to his fear of losing his son, named after him, and now the same age. Steve vehemently dismissed it, saying it was so long ago he hardly remembered it, and it had nothing to do with his current problems. He insisted he just wanted to focus on stopping his drinking and the affair.

Steve canceled the next session. When he returned the following week, he said he started thinking about his little brother and his tragic death. They had been throwing a ball around, when Steve deliberately threw it too hard, over Michael's head, laughing. Michael ran into the street to get it and was hit by a passing car. His parents were so distraught they never again talked about the accident, but Steve secretly blamed himself.

Here, the coincident timing of Steve's presenting concerns suggests the connection of his risky behavior and fears of causing loss with reactivation of his past loss experience. In a collaborative approach, when as therapists, we notice and wonder about a possible contributing influence, it's important not to impose our view. It is not our role to interpret clients' problematic situation, but rather to open and expand perspectives for them to consider. When a client initially rejects any connection, therapists should respectfully acknowledge that it may not be connected (as it may not). Yet we might suggest they keep in mind its possible relevance and sensitively broach it again when timely.

In presenting problems around separation, as when young adults leave home, we explore possible connections to earlier complicated losses in the family system. A future-oriented focus can sometimes be valuable, where a current crisis reactivates a past death and its repercussions for surviving family members, as in the following case:

Joanne and Ralph were seen in family consultation after their 22-year-old son, Joey, still living at home, survived a drug overdose on the eve of his wedding. In rehab, he was doing well, but Joanne was having panic attacks. She said it was harder for her to let him go than when their other children left home, but she didn't know why. Noting that Joey had been named after her, I asked about her own experience of leaving home and getting married. Joanne told of eloping against her father's strong objections. She was furious at his opposition, and he, in turn, refused to speak to her again. He died 8 months later of a heart attack without reconciliation. At this point in her story, Joanne became tearful and said, "Somehow it feels the same now."

It's important to inquire beyond the obvious dyadic relationship between Joanne and her father to explore other system patterns that might also be fueling her current distress. Joanne had been very close to her mother, who, once widowed, spent the rest of her life depressed and lonely. Asked if she ever worried that history might repeat itself, Joanne began to cry, saying she worried constantly about her husband's overweight and heart condition. In recent months, he had complained of chest pains but had refused to see a doctor. Joey's leaving to marry aroused her fear that something terrible would happen to Ralph and she would end up like her mother.

With Joanne's catastrophic expectations and her lack of a model for later-life marriage (Ralph's mother had also been widowed), the couple had never discussed any dreams after launching their children. Brief couple therapy focused on envisioning their future possibilities. Ralph had a medical workup and started to take better care of himself. They supported Joey's drug treatment and recovery, celebrated his wedding, and then took a "refresher honeymoon."

Striking accounts of extreme transgenerational anniversary reactions after violent deaths have been reported in early family systems studies (see Walsh & McGoldrick, 1991, 2004). When a child in the next generation reached the same age or developmental transition as the parent's traumatic experience, the young person suffered a mental health crisis, sometimes with violent acts. Byng-Hall (2004) described chilling situations in which traumatic death scenarios were replicated through a child's reenactment upon reaching the age of the parent at the time of the event. After one teenager tried to hang herself, it was learned that her mother, at the same age, had witnessed her brother's hanging death.

Such crises occurred in several families seen in my early clinical research (Walsh, 1983). One 15-year-old youth stabbed an adult stranger in the street in a dissociated episode, which was ignored by his parents. Following a repeated stabbing offense and psychiatric hospitalization, the family assessment revealed that the father, at age 15, had witnessed the stabbing death of his own father by a stranger in the street.

In another family (Walsh, 2016c), the father, a survivor of the Nazi Holocaust, never spoke of his or his family's experience, despite the camp numbers visible on his arm. His wife related that she had asked him once, when they first met, but he was so visibly shaken that she knew never to ask again. When their son turned 18, the father's gift to him was a summer trip to Europe, still without mentioning the horrific past experience. The son, on impulse, took a train to see a concentration camp. On route, he had a psychotic episode and was brought home and psychiatrically hospitalized. In my meetings with the family, the father acknowledged his earlier need to block all memories: at age 18, he had witnessed the shooting death of his brother, who had tried to stop soldiers from taking his parents away. He was deeply remorseful for his "thoughtless" gift to his son at the same age. In a follow-up contact a year later, the mother told me they had taken a family trip to the father's hometown in Poland, which was very healing—she also mentioned their son was now in college, majoring in communications.

Byng-Hall (2004) posited that such traumatic past experiences can become encoded in covert family scripts that may be out of awareness, particularly when communication about the events is blocked. Further study of such transgenerational anniversary patterns can increase our understanding of such disturbing systemic transmission processes. Therapeutic interventions aim to help clients gain awareness of covert patterns, to open blocked communication, and to differentiate present situations from the past so that history need not be repeated. Therapists can help them reappraise family history, replacing deterministic assumptions and catastrophic fears with an evolutionary perspective that integrates life experiences and yields meaning and hope for the future.

ADDRESSING COMPLICATED FAMILY DYNAMICS WITH LOSS

All family relationships have occasional conflict, mixed feelings, or shifting alliances. With a significant loss, painful emotions can be aroused for those who have experienced intense conflict, abuse or neglect, strong ambivalence, or estrangement. In those situations, it's important for clinicians to assess the family system and relational dynamics surrounding the loss to understand the meaning and context of presenting difficulties.

Perceived injustices and long-simmering hostilities in families often erupt in full force with a parent's death. Old family dynamics in sibling rivalries can be stirred up in the emotional intensity. Anger and bitterness may complicate grief and poison relationships for years to come. In one case, an adult brother and sister, fighting over a treasured photograph of their deceased mother, tore it in two. Furious at each other, they never spoke again (despite living in the same apartment complex) until coming to therapy 5 years later to repair their relationship so that their children could play together.

Sometimes survivors become enraged over felt injustices in a will and inheritance, which signify to them the meaning and significance of their bonds. One woman never forgave her father for leaving the family home and other property to her brothers; with traditional patriarchal views, he had always favored his sons. In one tangled stepfamily situation, after their father's death, the adult children from his first marriage filed a lawsuit against his widowed second wife, contesting his will that left most of his estate to her. They never forgave him for remarrying soon after their mother's death, and they treated her coldly, considering her a "gold digger." She was deeply pained: she had lovingly cared for him throughout his long illness, while his children had visited infrequently. Family mediation, sensitive to the complexities of divorce and stepfamily dynamics, was essential, combining individual and conjoint sessions toward reconciliation.

With the death of a troubled, abusive, or absent parent, grief can be especially fraught for survivors, affecting other relationships.

> Corinne came for therapy with a tangled knot of emotions 3 years after her father's death. Looking back, she was still furious about the glowing eulogies at his funeral. Her mother and brother and their relatives all knew he had been a "mean drunk" and treated his wife and children badly. But when she confronted them, they told her, "It's wrong to speak ill of the deceased. He was your father. Just remember the good times." She felt they invalidated her painful experience, leaving her isolated with intense, conflicting feelings and memories (see Chapter 7). She cut off all contact with her family, but it didn't help; she was drinking too much and regretted "taking it out" out on her husband, who didn't deserve her outbursts.

Complicated Loss and Past Relational Trauma in Presenting Problems

When a couple has suffered a pregnancy loss, well-intentioned family members and friends often encourage them to "try again" immediately, before they have emotionally processed their grief (see Chapter 7). In the following case, that loss was further complicated by self-blame connected to a traumatic loss that reactivated childhood relational trauma.

> Emma and Phil sought couple therapy because they were fighting over their inability to decide on the name for their baby girl, now 8 months old. The brief solution-oriented therapy ended "successfully" in a few sessions after the couple agreed on the baby's name. However, over the following month, Emma became increasingly depressed, unable to care for the infant, and one night took a handful of pills, wanting to take her own life.

Emma was referred to me for individual therapy. It was crucial to understand the meaning and circumstances of the baby's birth and her postpartum depression. Emma related that she became pregnant just 2 months after losing their much-desired first pregnancy, for which she blamed herself. We explored her earlier pregnancy loss experience more fully. At the sudden death of her stepfather, a "heavy drinker" who had sexually abused her in childhood, Emma had been overcome by a "crazy mix of emotions." Phil had suggested a relaxing weeklong getaway, where they both drank heavily. A month later, she was overjoyed to learn she was pregnant. When she suffered a miscarriage, she was devastated and blamed herself for her drinking binge. Urged by well-intentioned friends to have another baby right away to "get over" the loss, she found herself unable to attach to their new infant. When feeling pressed in therapy to name their daughter, they had decided on Carla, the same name she had planned for their first baby. She couldn't bear to hear the name and spiraled downward emotionally, becoming suicidal.

In later sessions, the therapist helped Emma to address painful childhood memories aroused by her stepfather's death and to assuage her self-blame in his abuse (common in survivors). She and her husband decided to give their daughter her own name, Miranda, and had the original name, Carla, carved on a stone, which they placed in their garden. With Phil's support, she found new joy in bonding with Miranda.

As in several cases above, we pay special attention to the significance of names and the naming of children in families. It's very common to name a child after a deceased loved one to honor that person and a cherished bond. Yet it's important to explore more complicated associations to a tragic or traumatic past loss situation.

Past Violent Death in the Context of Relational Trauma

When a violent death occurred in the context of ongoing relational trauma in childhood, posttraumatic difficulties for surviving loved ones can persist in deep fears of commitment, intimacy, and trust, as in the following case:

Rhonda came to therapy for help with her fears about getting married— she and her partner, Braden, deeply loved each other, but she had twice broken off their engagement. "I know he's faultlessly kind and considerate, but I just can't trust that he won't change and seriously harm me or any children we hope to have."

Rhonda carried catastrophic fears from her childhood. She had tried to lock away disturbing memories and had not shared them with

Braden. She realized it was time to unlock that vault. I supported her as she related all that had happened. On weekends her parents would go out drinking; upon their return, their escalating arguments would end in her father's physical abuse of her mother. Each time, Rhonda covered her head with pillows, trying not to hear the violence. Finally, the mother filed assault charges and received a protection order to keep him away from their home. When released from jail, furious at her legal action, he broke into the kitchen where they were making dinner. She watched as her father grabbed a butcher knife from the counter and hurled it at her mother, killing her baby brother, nestled in the mother's arms.

Here, the childhood witnessing of a violent death of a sibling, traumatic in itself, occurred in the context of recurrent relational trauma. In such cases, particular sensitivity, skill, and care are required in working with clients and in honoring their painful experience. A resilience-oriented, systemic trauma-informed approach (e.g., Barrett & Stone-Fish, 2014) is recommended. In the situation above, the therapist expanded the focus to the mother's resilient response: She took her children to safety to live with her extended family, where they remained well cared for and out of harm's way. The family took concerted action to gain the father's arrest, conviction, and sentencing for the heinous actions. Rhonda enlarged her view of the tragedy, with greater appreciation of her mother's nurturing and protection and of Braden's similar qualities of loving care.

Dilemmas in Therapy: To Tell or Not To Tell

In some cases, an impending death may pose troubling decisions that bring up long-buried secrets and reactivate painful memories of a past loss. Sometimes, clients come to therapy wanting the therapist to advise them what to do in a highly distressing predicament, as in the following case (Walsh, 2016c; see Figure 10.2):

Diane came for a consultation in an urgent family crisis. She and her husband, Dwayne, had raised their 16-year-old son, Jason, from birth and they enjoyed a happy family life. Jason did not know that Dwayne was not his biological father. Out of the blue, Diane had just received a phone call from Ron, her son's biological father. He told her he had terminal cancer and wanted to meet his son before he died. She asked me, "Should I tell Jason or not?"

It is not the therapist's role to resolve clients' dilemmas, especially on major life decisions that affect others. Rather, working collaboratively, I expanded our discussion to understand the situation more fully, to consider the options, and to support her meaning-making efforts to find her own pathway forward. Tearfully, she related the story. When Diane was in graduate school and in a serious relationship with Ron, she became pregnant. Ron, saying that he was not ready to raise a child, left her abruptly, moving across the country. She never heard from him again. For support, she turned to her close friend, Dwayne. Understanding her predicament, he assumed paternity, and they married before the baby was born.

It was helpful to unpack both sides of the dilemma and its complexities: what if she tells her son, and what if she does not? It was important to hear more about Jason and their family life in considering a decision. In the next session, Diane started by considering the ramifications of her preference not to tell. Jason was doing well in school and was enjoying his social life; his relationships with Diane and Dwayne were good. Learning the truth might be so upsetting that it could disrupt everything going well in his life and destroy his relationship with them. "Why rock the boat?"

I asked about Diane's own feelings about Ron contacting her with this request after all these years. She exploded in fury at his selfishness—the total lack of contact, support, or concern for Jason. "And for you?" I asked. Sobbing, she recalled the dreams she and Ron had shared for their future life together—how could he have abandoned her, pregnant with their child? She had tried to put that painful time out of her mind and just go on, making a new family with Dwayne. He was kind and generous, and he never brought up the past. "How could Ron wreck our family life

To Tell or Not To Tell

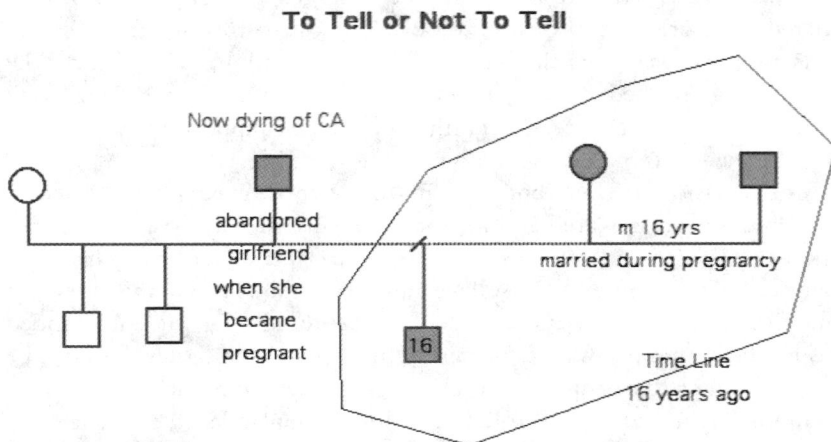

FIGURE 10.2. Genogram of family secret: Dilemma to tell or not to tell.

and ruin Jason's bond with Dwayne?!" "And what if he preferred his biological dad?" It was important to acknowledge her feelings and concerns as understandable in such a fraught situation.

In the next session, we explored the other option in her dilemma: the implications of telling Jason and revealing the secret. Diane had thought over the whole situation—now she realized the risks in *not* telling him. Ron had married and had children—what if they sought out Jason someday and he learned the truth—and that we had lied and prevented him from meeting his biological father before he died. He would hate us. And either way, the coverup of his paternity would come out.

Diane decided to tell Jason and offer him the chance to meet Ron. She felt it was the compassionate thing to do: to rise above her fears and past hurts. It also would convey her trust in Jason that he was strong and mature enough to handle the situation and trust that their family bonds were solid enough to weather the storms. We then considered the process of telling and the importance of talking it over first with Dwayne, and if he agreed, they'd do it together and would support his decision either way. Anticipating Jason's shock and upset, we brainstormed how they could "steady the family boat" though the turmoil—and his decision to visit Ron and meet his family. They agreed to tell Jason together and to hold each other through any upheaval. To be prepared, I asked how they thought Jason might react. She thought he might run off, but wouldn't do something destructive and would likely return. I encouraged her to keep a supportive openness to "hang in" with him through an immediate turbulent period.

Jason initially was disbelieving, then enraged at both parents. As predicted, he stormed out of the house. They called his best friend's parents and were reassured that he was there for the night. The next day he returned but refused to talk to them. The following day he asked for Ron's phone number. The parents told him they would support whatever decision he made. Jason decided to go to meet his father.

The visit was short but meaningful. Ron showed sincere remorse for having been so scared and immature in running out on Jason and his mother. He wanted Jason to know that he had just signed over part of his pension to contribute to his college fund. He said he knew this wouldn't erase the past, but he wanted to do what he could now. He commended Jason's mother and Dwayne for raising him so well (and after the visit, he wrote a long letter of apology to Diane). After returning home, Jason was grateful for his parents' confidence in him. I applauded their generosity in giving Jason and Ron this opportunity. Several months later, at Ron's death, Jason went to his funeral, and began connecting with his half siblings. Through this process, Diane's fear of losing their "intact" family was assuaged, as their bonds, while expanded, were strengthened by their trust.

This case also demonstrates how clinicians can address a dilemma around revealing hidden parentage when guided by a systemic approach, understanding varied perspectives, and coaching steps toward positive aims. Such dilemmas are becoming more common with advances in reproductive medicine, surrogacy in pregnancies, and popular DNA testing that reveals paternity. As clients grapple with their own particular situation, therapists need to be supportive of their decisions and pathways forward.

HEALING RELATIONAL WOUNDS AFTER A DEATH

Death ends a life but not a relationship, which continues on in the minds of survivors. Individuals often come to therapy long after the death of a significant family member still carrying painful wounds from the past. Some continue to be deeply troubled in ways that affect their lives and relationships with others. Some who had cut off contact or disconnected from painful memories find them surfacing in other contexts. Some, as in several of the cases described earlier, are jolted by unexpected arousal of long-suppressed memories and emotions by current crises in their lives. Many are remorseful that it is too late to repair grievances or to better understand a deceased parent. Most individual therapy models focus on the client's internalized images and problematic memories, which can reinforce a fixed view. Systemic therapists consider all individual views as inherently partial and subjective and therefore encourage clients to gain wider perspectives. Doing so does not disqualify one's own experience. Rather, it can enlarge understanding and contextualize troubling situations.

We may suggest that clients contact extended family members and others to clarify obscured information about a tragic death and loss. We encourage them to learn more about the life experience of a parent who is no longer alive. The most important element is respectful, genuine curiosity to understand loved ones and complex situations in their social and developmental contexts. In learning to ask questions and listen to others' views with an open heart, clients can reach fuller comprehension to bring coherence to their own experience. We encourage them to reconnect with important others at holidays, events, and reunions and to take active agency in planning and shaping family gatherings and sharing memorabilia. A *family life review* (see Chapter 4), can also be valuable, helping

surviving members to share different memories, to clarify misunderstandings, and to place hurts and disappointments in a larger context of life
challenges. Some questions may never be fully clarified, some ambiguities
may remain, and new information may open new questions. Yet, amid
complexity, we can help clients to recover caring aspects of troubled relationships and to update and renew relationships frozen in old conflicts.

Therapists can facilitate the process of reconnection with estranged
family members by coaching clients to repair cutoffs and conflicts and
to redevelop personal relationships with important family members who
are still alive. Because of the recursive nature of transactions in human
systems, changing one's own part in emotionally charged transactions can
interrupt vicious cycles, with change by others more likely to follow over
time. A genuine effort to understand others' positions and to strive for a
better relationship is the aim of differentiation. Whatever the response,
clients gain a more compassionate understanding of their own and others'
limitations and strengths.

It can be healing for clients to visit the graves of loved ones long
deceased or to return to their childhood hometown or places of special
significance. Rituals of remembrance and transformation can be healing,
even decades after a death. The use of journals and photos in therapy can
prompt storytelling about family members, relationships, and past events.
Letter writing to the deceased can be healing. Thoughtfully constructed
messages to surviving family members can aid in clarifying situations and
misunderstandings. Therapists can offer feedback on drafts to support clients' best efforts to express their pain, their caring for the other, and their
positive aims without attack, demandingness, or defensiveness. A difficult
message can be read and considered by the other without an immediate
defensive reply or counterreaction. Keeping a systemic perspective helps
clients to anticipate possible setbacks, understand them, and respond without reactive escalation.

The process of reconciliation in wounded bonds involves attempts to
incorporate disparate aspects of experience into a larger whole while giving each its place. It requires a shift in our perspective from a split view to a
larger, holistic perspective—from an "either–or" stance (If they hurt me so
badly, how could they have loved me?) to a "both–and" inclusive position:
(They loved me *and* they hurt me.) When clients reach out to other surviving members who are unable to respond as wished for, they have still
gained in generosity, and in a sense they reached for their best selves, true
to their ethical values (Fishbane, 2019). This facilitates greater acceptance
and enables them to embrace life with fuller integrity.

Even in cases of serious past injury or injustice, therapists can guide
repair of past relationships and healing of past emotional pain through

work toward restoration and forgiveness (Hargrave & Zasowski, 2016). Some cannot forgive a harm or injustice. Therapists need to respect each client's position. Where family members differ, it's important to help them respect each other's position. For those who choose to strive toward forgiveness, this work can be painful and difficult: It involves the intention and willingness to work toward repairing that relationship, even after severe damage. Forgiveness doesn't consist of simple platitudes or superficial statements that are expected to make the past go away. It is *not* intended to forget about serious harm. Rather, the aim is to forgive and remember. It provides the opportunity for accountability and compensation. When carefully guided, it can be unexpectedly fruitful.

Expanding Family Stories of Loss: Linking Past, Present, and Future

When working with clients from a resilience orientation, it is important first to listen to and honor their pain and suffering surrounding a loss. Without rushing to ease that distress, it's helpful to gradually enlarge the focus to show interest in their fuller life experience before and since the loss, with compassion for their struggles and with affirmation of their strengths and resources. Therapeutic inquiry can expand memories of painful loss to draw out the experience of resilience alongside suffering. Family stories and role models of adaptive coping can inspire current efforts. Therapists can help clients gain an evolutionary perspective that integrates painful losses and yields meaning and hope for the future. Time does not heal all wounds, but it does offer new experiences and vital connections that can help people gain new perspectives and forge new meaning and purpose in their lives.

Exploring a family's ancestry expands a sense of connectedness back through time and across generations. Some have a thin narrative of their family history, with little or no sense of their parents' earlier life experiences or of grandparents' lives before them. Looking back more broadly in family history can foster a broader contextual, evolutionary perspective. It's important to notice nuggets of resilience at times of past losses, as in a family's migration experience, enduring hardships and making their way in a new home. Stories of adversity are enlarged in drawing out the courage, perseverance, and inventiveness that enabled them to reorient and prevail. For clients who are struggling, reconnecting with the challenges and strengths of ancestors can be empowering (see Chapters 11 and 12).

In my work with Hope (see Chapter 1), readers will recall that she had lost her mother at age 7, then was sexually abused by her father, and just recently, in midlife, suffered the tragic death of her brother, her vital lifeline over the decades. She felt totally disconnected from her past. I encouraged her to learn more about her mother's family of origin and relatives whom she might connect with. She was energized in meeting two cousins and in learning that her great grandparents had been early settlers in her town. This prompted her to volunteer in her town's small historical museum, becoming involved in her community and finding meaning in deep connection to her family roots. No longer needing to hover anxiously over adult children's parenting, she enjoyed more satisfying bonds with them and her grandchildren.

Those who suffer early family trauma and loss cannot change the past, but they can learn from and grow out of that painful experience by loving others well. Their resilience involves coming to terms with painful loss experiences and integrating that meaningful understanding into current and future lives and relationships.

CHAPTER 11

Collective Trauma and Loss

Fostering Individual, Family, and Community Resilience

> Sorrow felt alone leaves a deep crater
> in the soul; sorrow shared yields new life.
> —*NOMATHEMBA* (the Zulu word for *hope*)[*]

Families and their communities are intertwined in the impact of catastrophic events and in the mobilization of their resilience. Complicated grief is common with the tragic loss of many lives, widespread devastation, and survivors' struggles to rebuild lives. Family functioning, vital social networks, and community services can be disrupted, especially with complex recurrent crises, ongoing stressors, and hardships such as food, housing, and income insecurity, with prolonged adverse conditions and insufficient resources. Therefore, in any intervention approach, it is essential to attend to the many losses suffered in family and community life and to support individual, interpersonal, and broader systemic efforts in rebuilding shattered lives (Denborough, 2012; Saul, 2013).

As discussed in previous chapters, mental health services can best foster recovery and resilience by reorienting attention from individual pathology to a multisystemic perspective. A resilience-oriented approach contextualizes the distress in the extreme adverse situation, addresses complicated grief, and facilitates individual, family, and community capacities for healing and positive adaptation. Table 11.1 summarizes the key processes in risk and resilience in traumatic loss situations.

---

[*]Drama recounting the tumultuous transformation from Apartheid in South Africa, by Ntozake Shange, Joseph Shabalala, and Eric Simon.

TABLE 11.1. Traumatic Loss: Key Family and Social Processes in Risk and Resilience

Vulnerabilities, risks for maladaptation	Facilitate key processes for resilience
Belief systems	
• Shattered assumptions; ambiguous or senseless loss • Sense of failure/fault; blame, shame, guilt • Hopelessness, despair; bleak outlook • Powerlessness: helpless, overwhelmed • Multigenerational legacy: trauma, losses, catastrophic fears • Spiritual distress; sense of injustice, punishment for sins; cultural/spiritual disconnection, void	1. Make meaning of traumatic loss experience • Normalize, contextualize distress. • Gain sense of coherence as shared challenge: comprehensible, manageable, meaningful. 2. Positive outlook: reorient, hope • Affirm strengths, build on potential. • Master the possible; accept what can't be changed. 3. Transcendent values; spiritual connection • Faith beliefs, practices, community; nature; arts • Purpose, meaningful pursuits; activism • Learning, transformation, growth
Organizational processes	
• Rigid, autocratic, or unstable—chaotic, unreliable, leaderless • Highly conflictual, or estranged bonds • Vital bond or role functioning lost: • Precipitous replacement • Unable to reallocate roles or reinvest in relationships • Socially isolated; unacknowledged or stigmatized loss • Institutional barriers; economic resources lost, unavailable	4. Flexibility to adapt and restabilize • Restore structure, routines, predictability • Reorganize; realign role functions • Strong leadership: coordination 5. Connectedness: family, social, and community • Lifelines; mutual support; social network • Repair estranged relationships 6. Economic and institutional resources
Communication/problem-solving processes	
• Unclarity about loss situation • Secrecy, denial of loss event • Blocked emotional sharing or high conflict • Gender constraints • Lack of appreciation, joy, respite • Blocked problem solving, decision making, or future vision	7. Clear, consistent information, messages • Clarify trauma and loss-related ambiguity. 8. Open emotional expression, empathic response • Respect individual, cultural differences. • Share pleasure, humor, respite amid sorrow. 9. Collaborative decision making, problem solving • Resourcefulness; build on small steps, successes • Proactive planning, preparedness; "Plan B"

This chapter focuses on the impact of devastating losses in major disasters; in the recent pandemic; in military combat, war-torn regions, and refugee experiences; in mass killings; and in the recent global pandemic.

TRAUMATIC LOSS IN MAJOR DISASTERS

Major disasters generally involve catastrophic conditions causing the loss of lives and widespread damage and disruption (Masten & Motti-Stefanidi, 2020; Parkes, 2008; Walsh, 2007). Environmental disasters, such as earthquakes, hurricanes, violent storms, flooding, drought, and wildfires, leave destruction in their wake. The distinction of natural versus human-caused disasters has blurred, with recognition of multiple intersecting factors involving human activity or negligence, as in global climate change and in accidents such as a plane crash, when many lives are lost.

> When a train derailed along Taiwan's coast, 51 people were killed (Qin, Chien, & Dong, 2021). After a sleepless night, grieving relatives gathered in the grim, painful task of identifying remains, emerging from the makeshift morgue shaken and distraught. Some discussed funeral arrangements and reviewed autopsy reports, while volunteers, Christian pastors, and Buddhist monks offered comfort. For some families, grief was complicated by frustration and ambiguity, unable to identify their loved ones, yet hoping DNA analysis would help.
>
> One survivor lost her husband and their son and daughter, both promising college students. Crawling through the smoke, she found their bodies under mangled wreckage. Her grief was compounded by self-recriminations as she struggled to understand the tragedy. She could not stop blaming herself for asking her children to go back to her ancestral home to see their grandparents and pay their respects. By chance, the family missed their train and a kindly ticket agent upgraded them to the Express. On board, she had sat at the back of the first car, while urging her husband and children to sit up front, which absorbed the greatest impact. "Why didn't I go sit with them?" she sobbed. Her survival and the seeming randomness of it all was unbearable.

As attention goes to comfort those who lost loved ones, those who survived the event themselves often become plagued by ruminations and survivor guilt. Others, unable to clarify the cause of a tragedy, have difficulty going on with their lives. Follow-up contact and sensitive exploration of meaning-making concerns are important.

When a school fire in Chicago took the lives of 95 children, bereaved families and the entire community were grief-stricken. Television news replayed horrific images of the scene and the removal of bodies, amplifying the distress. Year-long investigations into the cause shifted blame from to a smoker in the basement (later found innocent) to the school's locked emergency exits and to the city's systemic failures in safety inspections.

Several children who escaped the burning building were interviewed decades later about the impact on their lives (Shefsky, 2003). One child cringed when everyone kept telling her how brave she was. No one asked about her terrifying experience. She suffered silently, never revealing her deep guilt: in panic and the stampede to escape, she had clawed her way through the smoke-filled classroom, pushing aside classmates to reach the window. Another survivor, who suffered spinal injuries when she jumped, was welcomed home from the hospital as a hero by friends and neighbors; many, however, later avoided contact, uncomfortable at seeing her injuries, reminding them of the tragedy. Another survivor had lasting self-doubt from the inadvertent meaning she had taken from the message of the pastor who conducted the funeral. Intending to console the bereaved families, he said that God took his special angels. "Why didn't God choose me? Why wasn't I special?"

When a whole community suffers a widespread disaster, such as floods or wildfires, the multiple losses, dislocations, and adaptational challenges can be overwhelming: "It's a cascade of sorrows," as one survivor put it. Yet, in many places, what is remarkable is the determination of most to rebuild their homes, lives, and community because they value their bonds forged over time: their sense of belonging and deep roots matter above all else.

After wildfires tore through their community in Oregon, destroying thousands of homes, those who were suddenly homeless grappled with the dilemma: "Should we stay or go?" (Gardiner, 2021). Families in FEMA trailers, storage areas, and other temporary shelters had to rely on help from neighbors, relief organizations, and the state government. A year later, hundreds remained displaced.

One man recounted, "I can close my eyes and see everything around me on fire like that day. It was terrifying. When I got to the highway and turned around, my home was gone. We lost everything." A mother reported, "I have days where, out of the blue, I'll start crying. I just need to let it out. . . . Whenever I see black smoke I can't stop shaking." Another parent continued to have stomach pains, headaches, and trouble sleeping. The doctor told him that it was stress and to take it easy. But how could he rest: he had to keep looking for a house—finding nothing he could afford. Another father reported, "I try not to make my family feel sad. I never thought I would be in this situation, but I am hopeful I will find a place. Then we would try to heal ourselves from what happened to us."

They faced huge challenges in rebuilding their lives in a region with few affordable homes and a looming sense that more fires would come. Yet, unbreakable bonds kept them from leaving a community they felt bound to by work, school, and family ties. As one mother said, "If I go to another place I will be lost, more than I'm lost here." An 80-year-old woman said, "I looked around: no family, no nothing. It felt as though I had no connections to the universe, to the world. Insofar as I have any roots, they're here."

One resident, who came from Mexico 16 years earlier, shared his experience: "The valley, that's what made me stay. I said, 'Here's perfect.' Then I met my wife, Elva, and everything was perfect, like living in a dream. . . . We did a lot of work. When Grandpa and Grandma came, we had to add another room. Every day, I'd wake up and water my garden, pick up eggs, feed my chickens. . . . I want to rebuild. I want a little piece of property so we can come back. I don't want anything for free. I want a chance, for somebody to believe in us and say, 'OK, I'm going to lend you that money.' "

One mother lamented, "We may end up having to leave. I really want to stay. This community is amazing. The school has helped the kids tremendously since the fire. We have been doing everything we can to stay here because I wanted my daughter to graduate with her friends. Our house [was] where they always met, played games, listened to music, sat around bonfires." Another parent concurred, "Home is where families are. All my family is here. Everyone here was basically family. All the kids played together. I met my best friends here." Another added, "My life is here. Having to get up and move would be stressful all over again, like starting out from zero. A house is just a structure. Your home is the people."

As these poignant accounts reveal, the deep sense of rootedness, belonging, and connectedness in family, community life, and the place that becomes home can sustain determination to rise above tragic loss. Helping professionals can foster healing and resilience by understanding the impact and meaning of their clients' loss situation and both their immediate and long-term recovery challenges. Multifamily groups and community forums are valuable in mobilizing extended kin, social, and practical support in efforts to rebuild homes and lives.

Even small scraps of family life salvaged from the wreckage of a disaster can hold special meaning. When a tornado slashed through one Midwestern town, homes were ripped from foundations, with furniture and possessions scattered for miles. Residents in surrounding areas set up websites, posting photos of found items—a love letter, a child's doll, framed photos. One family found comfort in retrieving a vase—cracked but not shattered. It stands on the new mantelpiece in the home they are building on a more solid foundation.

More than surviving, resilience involves learning from a tragedy to rebound stronger, addressing the future needs of families and communities to thrive, as in community advocacy for affordable housing and jobs. Anticipation of future climate threats can spark creative visions and new legal requirements for more secure and environmentally attuned communities.

In disasters causing widespread destruction and a staggering toll of deaths, as in Turkey and Syria after the 2023 earthquake, survivors desperately tried to save each precious life they could. One Syrian woman, her mother, and brother were thankful to be pulled from the wreckage after 38 hours; however, her mother died of complications days later. After having survived the brutal Syrian conflict and lengthy refugee experience, this was too much to bear. The inaccessibility of essential aid and the failure of government rescue and recovery efforts compound the trauma, suffering, and prolonged displacement, as occurred after Hurricane Katrina. Too often in a disaster, those most affected—and neglected—are the most vulnerable and marginalized, especially those with limited means, the elderly, and with serious health problems (Norris & Alegria, 2005). For disaster preparedness and recovery, the need is critical for local, regional, and national emergency planning, coordination, communication, and follow-through. Families are often called the bedrock of a society; yet when disaster strikes, the lack of resources renders them vulnerable. The commitment to prevention and postdisaster planning for sustainable communities must prioritize policies and practices for resilient families.

LOSS AND RESILIENCE IN THE WAKE OF THE COVID-19 PANDEMIC

The lengthy COVID-19 pandemic has had profound and ongoing effects, with multiple losses and disruptions in lives (Walsh, 2020). In most disasters with a local, short-term crisis event, conditions gradually return to normal. But in this pandemic, the extreme conditions have had a global impact and an unpredictable roller-coaster course with a cascade of stressors and persisting adaptational challenges in the aftermath. It's important to understand and address painful experiences of multiple pandemic-related loss.

Addressing Complicated Grief in Traumatic Death Situations

In the grim statistics of the death toll, which climbed to unimaginable millions, we may lose sight of the suffering in each bereaved family, with emotional and functional impact radiating through relational networks (Stroebe & Schut, 2021). Many families lost cherished loved ones, and many lost essential resources in caregiving and financial security. The elderly and those with underlying medical conditions were at highest risk of death; yet COVID also took the lives of the young and healthy. Disproportionally high death rates also were incurred by low-income and racial/ethnic minority workers in jobs deemed essential (Watson, Turner, & Hines, 2020).

In severe cases of COVID-19, sudden medical crisis, hospitalization, and extreme physical suffering before death were excruciating experiences for patients, isolated in quarantine, and for their loved ones, isolated in their grief. Suffering was intensified when pandemic restrictions prevented family members from providing bedside comfort and sharing loving good-byes. Mourning was impeded by the limitations of funeral and burial gatherings. Both the dying and the bereaved were cut off physically from kin and social support.

> Amara, an Indian immigrant in her 40s, contacted me requesting telehealth therapy. She was in unrelenting anguish 10 months after her mother's death, in India, from complications of COVID. Her intense grief was complicated by her self-recriminations for the death.
>
> Amara's widowed mother was receiving care by their family doctor for a chronic heart condition. Before the pandemic, Amara would fly to India every few months to oversee her care and to cook her mother's favorite dishes. As the eldest sibling, she assumed primary responsibility for their mother. As pandemic travel restrictions persisted, she felt increasingly guilty that she couldn't tend to her mother's needs.
>
> Late one night, sound asleep, Amara received a call from the physician: her mother was suffering a medical crisis—he and her brother needed her to decide if she should be hospitalized. This was an agonizing dilemma, as the local hospital had many COVID patients, posing high risk of contagion. Alarmed by the urgent crisis, Amara told them to take the mother to the hospital. There, the overworked staff mistakenly put her in a COVID unit, where she contracted the virus and rapidly declined, requiring a ventilator over several weeks. Amara worried

constantly, feeling helpless at a distance. The medical ordeal was too much for her mother's heart, which failed just as she was recovering. Unable to join her family in funeral and cremation ceremonies, Amara felt isolated in unbearable grief and withdrew from her husband and her work. Her husband, initially understanding, was increasingly impatient for her to "return to normal."

As we explored the many facets of Amara's suffering, she said that the worst was blaming herself for the death by making "the bad decision." I acknowledged her excruciating dilemma: responsible for a sudden, critical life-or-death decision from afar. I suggested that she call the doctor to review the situation and hear his perspective. I also recommended a video call with her brother. In Amara's conversation with the physician, he acknowledged his own sense of urgency for hospital care, but also his hesitation, given the COVID risk. Yet, he said, either way, it was not possible for Amara to be there to attend to her, through no fault of her own. He told her he had long admired her devotion to her mother and knew the mother had valued her loving care before COVID intervened. "Her death is not your fault—it is this pandemic that took her life and has wreaked havoc on all our lives. We are all in mourning."

In the video call with her brother, Amara was nervous, believing that he blamed her for the death. In seeing her troubled face on the screen, he confessed his own sense of guilt for not keeping their mother safe in the hospital. Blaming himself for her death, he was struggling with his own inner turmoil. Amara and her brother began keeping weekly contact, consoling one another, and reminiscing about their childhood family life. They set up a memorial website, inviting stories and photos to honor their mother, and they planned a Zoom gathering to celebrate her life. While Amara had occasional days of deep sadness in missing her beloved mother, she increasingly reengaged in her family life and career.

Addressing Multiple Pandemic-Related Losses

In the ripple effects of the lengthy pandemic, many families experienced multiple losses and an ongoing, pervasive sense of overload and disorientation (Walsh, 2020). Parents struggled to manage job and childrearing demands when schools and daycare centers were shuttered. Many lost jobs and financial security. Those with the least resources suffered the most daunting challenges in moving forward. Longstanding socioeconomic and racial disparities in the United States heightened pandemic-related risks for disadvantaged and marginalized communities. Pandemic-related aftershocks have continued to disrupt lives and threaten recovery efforts.

Many are grappling with the loss of pre-crisis ways of life and the threatened loss of future hopes and dreams. Most widespread is the loss of a sense of normalcy in shattered assumptions about our lives and connections with the world around us. With the future unpredictable, many are navigating a roller-coaster course, anxious and exhausted.

The emotional, relational, and functional toll of pandemic-related challenges has been overwhelming for many and has exacerbated preexisting struggles for some. The demand has surged for both adult and youth mental health services. There has been an alarming increase in road accidents, murders, suicides, and addiction-related deaths (see Chapter 9), with an urgent need for family involvement in prevention efforts and in bereavement counseling. Meeting the mental health needs of healthcare and emergency personnel should also be a priority. Most worked tirelessly with an overload of medical crises and tended to dying patients, their own needs unattended.

This pandemic has affected us all. In the aftermath, therapists should anticipate that many who suffered losses will seek counseling much later, sometimes presenting other problems. Some who contended with multistress challenges suppressed their pain to carry on. Most were exhausted by the long ordeal and eager to plunge ahead with postponed plans, new ventures, and simple pleasures in life—a common and understandable desire. Other urgent matters also come to the fore, from personal, family, and financial matters to societal and global concerns. In a society that minimizes loss, the bereaved may also feel social pressure to move on, their grief disenfranchised (see Chapter 7). "No one wants to see our sadness," said one woman who lost her husband and sister to COVID. Those who submerged their suffering may need help later with the reverberations of loss in their lives going forward (see Chapter 10). This requires pacing of interventions attuned to each situation, weaving in attention to grief, emerging challenges, and future directions. Efforts will be needed both for restoring or modifying valued continuities and for reenvisioning possibilities for adaptive change and the ability to thrive.

TRAUMATIC LOSS IN WAR AND CONFLICT REGIONS

The tragic toll of death and loss in military combat and in regions directly affected by armed conflict require mental health and psychosocial support services to those in distress. Strength-based, systemic approaches foster both individual and family healing and resilience, addressing immediate and long-term challenges.

Traumatic Loss and Moral Injury in Military Service

Over the past two decades, with post-9/11 wars and multiple deployment of troops in Iraq and Afghanistan, American military service personnel have suffered a rising incidence of PTSD, depression, substance abuse, violence, divorce, and suicide. Shockingly, more lives of service members and veterans have been lost to suicide than to combat deaths. While relational or financial stresses are factors in some cases, more often, deaths by suicide and other self-harm behaviors are associated with chronic debilitating service-related medical conditions, traumatic brain injuries, PTSD, depression, and opioid use for pain relief. One war veteran, in a support group after heavy drinking and reckless driving in a suicide attempt, described his horror and helplessness when his platoon members were killed or badly wounded by an improvised explosive device. The worst was seeing the shattered body of his closest buddy—the "only real friend" he had. He suffered flashbacks and paralyzing shame for not being injured or not being able to save him.

Recent studies suggest that service members and veterans who experience moral injury—distinct from PTSD—have the highest risk of suicide (Griffin et al., 2019). *Moral injury* concerns an anguished sense of unworthiness that derives from violation of deeply held psychological, cultural, and spiritual mores. Damage to moral belief systems occurs through participation in conduct that violates one's deepest human values, producing deep shame, guilt, and self-loathing. Such incidents might involve betrayals of trust in actions, or failure to act, in situations of extreme violence or torture, within-rank "friendly fire," or sexual abuse. The death of civilians, especially women and children, is especially hard to bear.

Suicide prevention is hampered by the stigma and potential negative career consequences of reporting emotional distress for service personnel and long waitlists for veterans' mental health services. When atrocities are denied, minimized, or dehumanized as "collateral damage" by the military, as in "mistaken" drone strikes, it takes enormous courage to acknowledge them. Profound shame and guilt involving acts of inhumanity leave service members feeling morally unfit to reenter the human community, to receive praise and awards for their valor, or to have intimate relationships. After experiencing something unspeakable, how do you trust again, yourself or others, or accept the love of a spouse, children, or parents? As one veteran asked, "How do you look at your child when you murdered a child?"

The predominant treatment models for combat-related trauma have been individually based and focused on reducing symptoms of PTSD and related mental disorders. A resilience-oriented systemic framework situates the many varied facets of the traumatic experience, including the spiritual (moral) dimension, in the extreme conditions of war and combat. It contextualizes intense anguish as a normal, human reaction to abnormal and inhumane conditions and actions.

Litz, Liebowitz, Gray, and Nash (2016) developed a research-informed psychotherapy framework based on adaptive disclosure to guide practice in addressing military trauma, loss, and moral injury. They urge clinicians to sensitively explore such wounds, which may be a source of despair, isolation, destructive behavior, and risk of self-harm. Past events cannot be undone, but adaptive healing involves a journey of remorse and forgiveness, with attempts to make reparations to survivors, if possible, and going forward, with actions to prevent suffering and loss for others.

One chaplain advised a veteran unable to forgive himself for having mistakenly opened fire on a family, killing five children. The chaplain asked, "Can you go out and find five children at risk you might help to thrive?" In response, the vet became involved in mentoring children in Big Brothers/Big Sisters and became active in a veterans' organization working to prevent war atrocities. Recent studies have pointed to the value of programs for veterans' teamwork on community projects—for example, rebuilding homes and creating parks in blighted neighborhoods. Such programs provide comradeship on a positive mission and purpose that revives their sense of connectedness and worth.

The family impact of combat-related trauma was first studied among World War II and Vietnam War veterans. Research has documented the psychological, spiritual, and relational effects on the military spouses and children of service members' traumatic stress related to their war-zone deployments, combat exposure, and postdeployment difficulties. Secondary traumatization can occur through ongoing transactions in couple and family life with disruptive symptoms, withdrawal, or harmful behaviors (Catherall, 2004; Figley, 2002). Research finds the positive influence of family resilience processes in mitigating negative effects (MacDermid, 2010). Resilience-based interventions address stresses, strengthen bonds, and facilitate family support for a returning service member's resilient adaptation to life (e.g., Saltzman, 2016). Workshop and weekend retreat formats help families navigate pre- and postdeployment challenges and foster healing from injuries, trauma, and losses as they revitalize family relationships and reenvision future possibilities.

Traumatic Loss and Resilience in War-Torn Regions

Loss is a central issue for almost all persons displaced by conflict or disaster, requiring greater attention in helping children and adults in great distress (Jones, 2020). International humanitarian aid groups caution to avoid misapplication or overdiagnosis of PTSD and to understand the varied reactions, family and social influences, and cultural meanings of deep anguish. While most do not suffer long-term trauma effects, massive losses and displacement interfere with mourning processes and impact physical, mental, and relational well-being. Therefore, it is vital to understand complex loss situations and to facilitate culturally appropriate processes for healing and resilience.

Family life can be shattered in the vast human toll and devastation wrought by war; violent ethnic, tribal, religious, and political conflicts; and genocidal campaigns. Family members may be forcibly separated, kidnapped, or made to witness the brutal killing and abuse of loved ones. Young boys and girls may be pressed into combat, enslaved, or sold in sex trafficking. Efforts to trace those missing or displaced and reconnect those separated with their families can be vital in their resilience. The comfort and security provided by warm, caring relationships is critical in withstanding trauma for populations affected by war, including social and personal uprooting, family disruption, separation and loss, mental and physical suffering, and vast social change. The security provided by families in war zones buffers such stresses as bombings, air raids, and the horrors of witnessing violent death (Masten & Narayan, 2012).

In 1998–2000, our Center in Chicago co-designed resilience-based multifamily groups for refugees who fled ethnic cleansing campaigns in Bosnia and Kosovo (Walsh, 2016c; Weine et al., 2003, 2004). That led to a multiyear partnership in Kosovo between Kosovar mental health professionals and a team of American family therapists (the Kosovar Family Professional Educational Collaborative). Community-based, resilience-oriented, family-centered training and services were developed to enhance local capacities to meet the overwhelming service needs in the war-torn region (Becker, Sargent, & Rolland, 2000; see Chapter 12).

Where communities in underresourced regions of the world have suffered poverty, war, and conflict across decades and generations, violence, loss, and despair can fracture family functioning, affecting couple bonds, parenting, and child well-being. Collaborative systemic approaches promote recovery and resilience (Landau, 2007; Landau, Mittal, & Wieling, 2008; Saul, 2013). In situations of complex trauma, resilience-oriented approaches emphasize the importance of fostering a meaningful vision of the future; the experience of being valued and valuing others; hope of a better world and life worth living; feeling empowered (versus helpless); and collaborative efforts to create workable solutions (Barrett & Stone-Fish, 2014).

TRAUMA, LOSS, AND RESILIENCE
IN DISPLACEMENT AND REFUGEE EXPERIENCES

As the Afghanistan government fell in August 2021, Haris Tarin, a founder of the Afghan-American Foundation, described his experience aiding the wave of refugees fleeing the Taliban takeover (Fadel, Jarenwattananon, & Hodges, 2021). Thirty years earlier, in the Soviet invasion, with over a million people killed, he had escaped with his family, and after an arduous journey, they had resettled in the United States. He and older Afghans were now reliving that trauma, watching it happen again. He described the immense fear of Afghans caught in the current crisis. People lost everything overnight, fleeing with a small sack and a few photos or memorabilia.

NPR interviewer, Leila Fadel, asked about the resettlement experience, noting that most stories we hear are about getting to safety—but very few are about what it must be like to leave your entire life and your homeland behind.

"The resettlement experience is difficult—I remember it as a child . . . the pain of my father, when he found out, just a couple years after he settled in the U.S., that his mother died, then his sister died, and his brother died. And there was this constant feeling of guilt—of survivors' guilt—that we made it through, but our families didn't, and they continued to suffer. And having to relive that again, twice in one lifetime, is extremely painful and traumatic for so many people.

"And the children I have seen, I can see it in their eyes, I can see it in the eyes of the mothers who are crying and the fathers who don't know what type of life they'll be able to provide for their children. And so the mothers and the fathers are constantly asking, 'Will my children be OK?'"

The interviewer asked, "What do you tell them?" Tarin replied:

"All I can do is provide my personal experience. I can't make any promises to them. But I can say I've gone through it; I know how it feels. I can hold them. And I can tell them I ended up being OK and my family ended up being OK even though we struggled and so will you."

Asked if there was a particular incident that stood out in helping people, he replied, "One of the refugees I met actually gave me his last piece of gum. He said, 'I want you to keep this with you—to remember that you helped out. This is our land and I'm not leaving it by choice.' And he took the wrapper and gave me the gum and he said, 'This is something that will bind us through this process.'"

Lengthy wars in Syria and Ukraine have displaced over half the population. Untold numbers are missing or displaced in conflicts worldwide.

In addition to the heartbreak of loved ones killed in brutal assaults, surviving family members must endure painful separations, elders and others left behind, and an uncertain future. In the chaos, deadly threats, and mass displacement, there is heightened anxiety with ambiguous losses (Boss, 2017; see Chapter 7). Many are desperate for information to learn if loved ones are alive and safe and to restore contact, however possible. Yet, the human capacity for resilience emerges in the active resistance and creative strategies of underground networks, such as those in Afghanistan to educate girls despite death threats. In Ukraine, the strong government leadership and cohesive sense of national unity and cultural pride motivate all efforts to repel the invasion and restore their homeland. Despite ongoing terror and destruction, artists and musicians from bombed out towns find new shelter and use social media to bring light and hope to audiences, energizing their collective spirit of resilience.

Refugees face myriad challenges in overcoming experiences of physical and psychosocial trauma and loss, with further privation, separations, and relocations in migration. Abduction, starvation, torture, rape, imprisonment, and dehumanizing treatment are all too common. Many have suffered multiple traumatic experiences with bombings or brutal torture and killing of loved ones and the loss of homes and communities. Many face lengthy stays in camps for refugees or internally displaced persons, as in the Zaatari camp for Syrian refugees in Jordan, where over 80,000 adults and children have been living in limbo, some for a decade, unable to return home or to their former lives. With the support of governmental and nongovernmental organizations (NGOs), community services have been set up to meet essential needs, such as clinics, classrooms, and play areas for children. While they cannot control their future fate, they practice small acts of resilience in their everyday lives. People have set up food stalls and small shops to meet residents' needs as they forge makeshift communities. In the walled camp and bleak desert surroundings, residents painted the outside wall of a community center with a vibrant landscape of fertile fields, forests, and mountains, as a hopeful vista.

Many who have fled the country must move from place to place in seeking asylum and may suffer further separation in transit from a loved one, close companion, or cherished pet. With resettlement, the focus of social services is primarily on practical adaptational challenges and acculturation to a new way of life. It's crucial that helping professionals sensitively explore the painful loss of loved ones and lives left behind in migration and help to restore connections for resilience in going forward (Falicov, 2014).

Ahmed, a 24-year-old Syrian asylum seeker in Germany, sought therapy, saying, "Life is more than I can bear." He seemed to be doing well in resettlement, studying German and working diligently to pay for lodging with a roommate. The therapist asked to hear what troubled his mind. He replied that his sister had called him from Syria to inform him that his mother had died after an illness. The family hadn't told him earlier because they didn't want to cause him more upset, since he couldn't legally return home to see her. He was angry not to have been told that she was ill, and he felt helpless so far away, unable to comfort her or search for a treatment to save her life. Had he known she was dying, he would at least have called her to convey his love one last time. He sobbed, "She meant everything to me; she was always there for me. Now that's she's gone, I don't know how to go on living."

Over the following weeks, the focus of therapy sessions broadened to explore Ahmed's past life and migration experience. He had been a college student when his world came apart. His father, arrested for his political views, died in prison. Shortly after, he took part in student anti-government protests and was jailed. Ahmed paused, anxious and uneasy about continuing his account. With the therapist's encouragement, he revealed that he had been brutally sexually assaulted in jail. Upon release, he fled into Turkey. Finding no future prospects there, without legal rights to study or work, he decided to seek asylum in Europe. The passage across the sea to Greece, on rickety boats, was treacherous. Passengers were sold fake lifejackets filled with newspaper. In rough waters and the darkness of night, a woman and the child in her arms were swept overboard and drowned. When the boat, reaching shore, broke up on the rocky shoals, he was grateful that local fishermen rescued survivors.

Ahmed next recounted his perilous journey through Eastern Europe, fearful of being detained and jailed. At a bus stop, when overheard speaking Arabic to another passenger, he was dragged away and beaten by local men. Asked how he had found the strength to continue, he replied that a kind motorist picked him up and took him to his home. The family welcomed him, cleaned his wounds, and gave him dinner, a bed for the night, and fresh clothes, with their encouragement for the journey ahead.

Ahmed's therapist, showing compassion in learning all he had endured, remarked on his courage and perseverance in his efforts to forge a new life. Ahmed breathed deeply. Quiet for a while, he reflected that he didn't do it alone. He prayed daily to God for strength. And he was grateful for the generosity of the motorist and his family. "I need to remember that there's more love and goodness in the world than hate and brutality. That's what my mother always taught me." He took a small photo of his mother out of his wallet, saying, "She was the one who encouraged me to flee to safety and make a new life. Even when she wasn't with me on that journey, I always had her photo to keep her close with me." This led him to realize that her spirit was still with him, and he still had her photo, her love, her memory, and all she taught him to guide him forward in life.

TRAUMATIC LOSSES IN VULNERABLE COMMUNITIES AND IN MASS KILLINGS

Recurrent violence and traumatic deaths take a terrible toll in marginalized communities, disproportionally affecting low-income and racial, ethnic, and religious minorities. Worldwide, LGBTQI+ people face violent attacks, imprisonment, torture, and even death simply because of who they are or who they love.

The frequency of traumatic deaths can become a common shock. Yet, a pervasive sense of loss and dread wound the mind, body, and spirit of all children and adults who live with recurrent threat to their lives and loved ones (Weingarten, 2004). With the proliferation of guns in the United States, lethal violence takes a tragic toll, too often in low-income communities of color (see Chapter 9). In the grim statistics, no one feels secure: Parents worry if their child will make it home safe. As one mother sadly observed, "We never know who will be with us or lost tomorrow." Some who have lost close friends or family members try to numb the recurrent pain, terror, and helplessness with alcohol or drugs or by shutting off emotions and concern about themselves or others.

The disproportionate police killings of Black, Indigenous, and other persons of color, often resulting from racial profiling and misguided law enforcement, shatter the community's trust in those charged with providing protection. There is understandable outrage at the further injustice that comes with lack of accountability or meaningful reforms.

When we think of "community violence," it is imperative not to blame the community, assume the worst of its residents, and write off their potential to thrive. Families and entire communities suffer from the impact of systemic barriers and ongoing stressors of poverty, lack of resources, racism, and discrimination (Hardy, 2023). Contending with disrespect and blighted conditions, most families show remarkable courage in living their daily lives, striving to raise their children well to give them a better future. Changes in larger systems and socioeconomic structures are essential for families and communities to thrive.

At the local level, programs involving families and community mentors develop empowering relationships with youth who are at high risk of gang involvement and encourage strivings for positive development (Gorman-Smith, Henry, & Tolan, 2004; Walsh, 2016a). Neighborhood-based programs, such as Take Back the Streets, build collective resilience, as they combat violent crime by bringing together residents, police, and social agencies to work collaboratively and build a sense of pride and empowerment.

Surviving family members need ongoing support and advocacy. Many experience further distress in lengthy, convoluted processes in the criminal justice system. Most are better able to go on with their lives when they feel that justice has been served. Families of offenders are too often neglected by mental health and justice professionals. Parents commonly face social condemnation with presumptions of blame. Grounded in a deep conviction in the worth and potential of an offender, movements for restorative justice involve families and their communities in concerted actions.

Confluence of Historical and Ongoing Trauma, Loss, and Resilience

In the United States, Black, Indigenous, and other communities of color have suffered multiple, recurring traumatic experiences of oppression and loss across generations. From our country's founding, the removal and annihilation of Native American tribal communities and the enslavement of African Americans left brutal legacies of racism across the centuries that continue to our present times.

In the painful history of Indigenous boarding schools in North America, children were taken from their families and communities and stripped of their cultural and spiritual roots in efforts to "civilize the savage." Children who died were buried in secret unmarked graves; those who survived suffered routine violence. Many survivors forged resilience by showing resistance and by reclaiming their identity and connections, as in the following account (Callimachi, 2021):

> For decades, Ms. Smith barely spoke Navajo. From her first day in the school, she never again practiced the morning prayer after her brutal beating. They took away her name and language when they took her clothing and moccasins and cut her hair. She thought she had forgotten them, until years later, working at a hospital, a Navajo couple came in with their dying baby and she found that the words she thought had been beaten out of her were still there. Looking back, she recognized small but meaningful ways she had resisted—doing the traditional prayer "in my heart." She now makes jewelry with traditional elements, like "ghost beads" from dried juniper berries. In selling them online, she chose her birth name, *Dzabahe*, whose Navajo meaning endured: "woman who fights back."

In our therapeutic efforts with those who are struggling in their lives, we need to bear witness to stories of suffering and loss, and we also need to support clients in deepening connections with cultural and spiritual resources that can nourish their resilience (Falicov, 2016; Kirmeyer, Dandeneau, Marshall, Phillips, & Williamson, 2011). In working with Black clients, Ken Hardy (2023) stresses the need for therapists to recognize the role of transgenerational trauma in the suffering and struggles that they bring to therapy. Life-altering and debilitating racial trauma and traumatic loss have affected countless numbers. A confluence of historical and persistent experiences of discrimination and social and economic inequity devastate one's sense of self—emotionally, psychologically, physically, and relationally—while also depleting strategies for coping. Elaine Pinder-hughes's (2004) exploration of her African American family's transgenerational legacies of loss enriched her clinical work with Black families (see Chapter 12). Yet, she also stresses that the consequences of generations of trauma, terror, injustice, exploitation, and disenfranchisement over 400 years cannot be changed substantially by individual therapies and medication alone. Interventions must address the interwoven impact of past and ongoing trauma and loss in personal lives with the complex operation of racism in maintaining their vulnerability. Understanding their confluence is necessary for transformative societal policies that will address problems of invalidation, discrimination, poverty, exclusion, segregation, and socioeconomic disparities.

Casualties in Mass Killings

Mass killings are no longer unthinkable events, with the growing epidemic of mass shootings in the United States targeting schools, houses of worship, workplaces, and public spaces. After each horrific event, as the rest of the world moves on, loved ones carry an unspeakable sorrow commingled with outrage at the availability of assault-style weapons that produce such carnage and at gun control legislation that is repeatedly blocked. Families of the deceased and the children and adults who narrowly survive the shootings need help as they struggle to find their own paths in their grief. Their growing activism has been galvanizing wider public support for preventive mental health services and larger systemic changes.

In this age of widespread insecurity, with threats by domestic and foreign terrorists and right-wing militia groups, we are all living in a more volatile and insecure environment. Case studies of group recovery have found that catastrophic events, traumatic loss, and suffering sometimes lead to a breakdown in community morale and stagnation of future development. Yet when governmental actions are responsive, it fuels resourcefulness—rather than helplessness—and sparks new purpose and growth. Amid the anguish after mass casualties, remarkable demonstrations of community resilience emerge when local people come together in outreach to aid those who have been directly impacted. Professionals, volunteers, and rescue workers join forces in providing effective crisis intervention for those in urgent need and a strong support system to meet the many needs of survivors in the aftermath. This process of collaboration, meaning making, and active agency in response to the traumatic experience fosters their resilience (Walsh, 2016c). Rituals of remembrance promote unity and healing in the community through meaningful and life-affirming gatherings that honor the lives lost and instill faith in the long recovery process. Multifamily groups, community forums, and networks of parents, educators, and counselors are valuable to share experiences, respond to concerns, provide information and mutual support, and mobilize concerted action for individual and collective healing and resilience.

FOSTERING HEALING AND RESILIENCE IN COLLECTIVE TRAUMA AND LOSS

Psychosocial support interventions are vital in the immediate aftermath of catastrophic events for all who have suffered trauma and loss. Relieving acute distress and mobilizing resources can be crucial to prevent more serious and complicated grief. Crisis intervention can be immensely helpful in providing initial information and services. Helpful guidelines on parenting practices can promote child adjustment (Girwitz, Forgatch, & Wieling, 2008; Jones, 2020). Unhelpful are single-session debriefing programs that focus narrowly on individual trauma symptoms and open overwhelming and painful emotions, including helplessness and rage, without follow-up and family and social support (Emmerik, Kamphuis, Hulsbosch, & Emmelkamp, 2002).

Shared Beliefs and Practices in Family and Community Resilience

When catastrophic events occur, survivors cannot return to normal life as they knew it. Rather than the common image of resilience as "bouncing back," we might better view it as "*bouncing forward*" to adapt, over time, to an uncertain future (Walsh, 2002). Shared facilitative beliefs shape experience and pathways in adaptation for family and community resilience (see Chapter 2). Helping professionals can foster efforts: (1) to *make meaning* of the crisis and ongoing challenges; (2) to (re)gain a *hopeful outlook* that supports active agency; and (3) to transcend personal suffering and hardship through larger values, connections, and practices.

Meaning making and recovery involve grappling to understand what has been lost, how to cope and adapt, and how to prevent future tragedy. Hope is most essential in times of despair, fueling energies and efforts to cope and to rebuild lives. Perseverance, flexibility, and ingenuity are essential to navigate complex and changing situations, particularly when the future is precarious. More than surviving painful losses and managing stressful conditions, the suffering and struggle can yield personal and relational transformation and growth. Events of great magnitude sharpen awareness of the fragility of life; with time and shared reflection, they can spark reappraisal of what matters most going forward. Time does not heal all wounds, but it offers new perspectives, experiences, and connections that can help people to adapt and thrive.

Over the ages, individuals, families, and communities have shown that, in coming together, they could endure the worst forms of suffering and loss, and with time and concerted effort, rebuild and grow stronger. Overwhelming tragedy can bring out the best in the human spirit: ordinary people show extraordinary compassion and generosity in helping kin, neighbors, and strangers. In active coping efforts and in reaching out to others, people build resources that they may not have tapped otherwise. In the wake of devastating losses, the bereaved cannot bring back deceased loved ones and may not recover all that was valued, yet their suffering and struggle can yield deeper bonds, meaningful life priorities, and new purpose.

Intervention Principles to Support Healing and Resilience

Resilience-oriented interventions are most helpful when they (1) contextualize distress; (2) draw out strengths and active coping strategies for empowerment; (3) mobilize family and social support for ongoing recovery; and (4) offer follow-up sessions, as well as more intensive mental health services for those in severe and persisting distress. Music, artwork, drama, play therapy, journals, and guided activity books can be valuable resources, especially with children, adolescents, and families (Gil, 2014; Kliman, 2007). Interactive tools can help them express their experience of suffering and promote their emotional processing and resilience after traumatic events. Drawing, coloring, and word activities can help children remember, document, and make sense of their experience, integrating sad, bad, and scary parts, with helpful, brave, and good things people did. Older youths can describe in journals what they learned; what would be helpful now; and things that they, their families, and their community could do to rebuild and to be more prepared in the future.

In all interventions, including brief approaches, it is important to understand family grief and adaptational processes over time. Directly affected families often show an initial drop in functioning; some say they "hit rock bottom." Over the following months, most families experience a roller-coaster course in efforts to cope and adapt with a pileup of loss-related stressors and other family crises. Many, however, rise above past baselines, achieving higher levels of family functioning and growth. Families often gain resilience through efforts in meaning making, tapping spiritual resources, open emotional expression, and collaborative problem solving. For families to thrive, it is also essential to bolster social supports and economic resources.

The long and varied paths in healing emotionally and in rebuilding lives require a longitudinal perspective to address emerging stressors and adaptational processes over time, with the flexible availability of professionals and agencies. Survivors frequently note that there were times when they suffered so deeply that they didn't know if they could face another day, or they felt that life no longer had meaning; yet a loved one or friend supported them in rallying to carry on. It can be devastating for those unable to save loved ones who perished. One man was distraught that he wasn't able to rescue his wife from their burning apartment building. Still, her last words kept him going: "Take care of the kids." He said, "It's hard every day; I've never had to do this before. I didn't know how—but I'm finding I can do it. I hear her voice, and it gives me the strength and determination."

In the press of immediate practical demands, family members may suppress emotional needs or thoughts of painful losses. Many only seek counseling months later, after initial social support wanes and distress intensifies with the full impact of losses and emerging challenges. This requires pacing of interventions and follow-up sessions, weaving in attention to grief, emerging challenges, and future directions, and allowing time for respite and replenishment of energies.

As studies of resilience amply document, in struggling through hardship, reaching out to others, and making active coping efforts, people tap resources they may not have drawn on otherwise and gain new abilities and perspectives on life. Each survivor's experience is unique, yet the human compassion and generosity that frequently emerge are remarkable. In the widespread Ebola outbreak in West Africa, one physician noted that amid the horrible deaths in the isolation wards, there were moments of grace. Mothers whose babies had died would feed and care for infants who were orphaned.

Another disaster can reactivate past trauma but also offer opportunities for further healing. Families of those who died in the terrorist-caused plane crash over Lockerbie, Scotland, in 1988 found their pain revived by another plane crash 8 years later—one father described it as "like a scab torn off a deep wound." Yet, many of the Lockerbie families came forward to offer support to the recently bereaved families, finding that their assistance furthered their own long-term recovery.

Extensive work with refugees has found an intricate relationship between connections to the environment and the healing of mind and body; in experiencing beauty or social connection, neurochemical processes are activated that literally begin to heal psychic wounds. As family, friends, colleagues, and community groups can provide connectivity, nature and the arts can provide beauty and renewal in the wake of loss.

Multilevel Systemic Approaches in Healing and Resilience

Traumatic losses reverberate throughout families and their communities; in turn, their collective response can help or hinder recovery. Catastrophic events can awaken us to what really matters in life and inspire us to reorder our priorities and take the initiative in caring actions to benefit others. Communities have shown that they could endure the worst forms of suffering and grief and yet, with time and great effort, rebuild and grow stronger.

In humanitarian crises, multisystemic resilience-oriented approaches draw on and expand individual, family, and community resources, as well as their recursive synergy, as critical components of positive adaptation after widespread trauma and loss (Masten, 2019). Best practices share common principles: (1) helping professionals identify and partner with local resources to assess individual, family, and community needs and both available and needed resources; (2) outside professionals take a consultative role, supporting local leaders and building capacity in training and services to establish a matrix of healing responses from psychosocial support to more intensive mental health services (Landau, 2007; Saul, 2013). Through best practices of global humanitarian relief efforts, similar principles are advocated for resilience-oriented approaches in mental health and psychosocial support (International Medical Corps, 2017; Whitney, 2016).

In response to experiences of traumatic loss, systemic approaches highlight five themes in resilience-oriented interventions:

1. Building individual, family, and community capacities and enhancing social connectedness as a foundation for recovery by strengthening social support systems; by coalition building; and by sharing information, resources, problem solving, and prevention.

2. Sharing stories, validation, and destigmatizing of the trauma experience to encompass varied experiences and both the struggle and resilience in coping and adaptation.

3. Encouraging family and community members with diverse skills, talents, and ages to contribute to the community's resilience. Elders may bring stories, lessons, and coping strategies from their life experience and survival of past adversity, as the young renew capacities for play and creativity.

4. Reestablishing the rhythms of life and engaging in collective mourning and healing ceremonies and through the expressive arts and music.

5. Promoting collaborative meaning making, renewed hope, and active efforts toward a positive future vision in rebuilding and transforming lives.

In the wake of tragic events, remarkable resilience emerges in the many stories of courage and endurance and inventive strategies in coping and adapting. Through crisis, trauma, and suffering a creative process arises from the synergy of members coming together to work toward a common purpose. Resilience-oriented practice approaches help families and communities expand their vision of what is possible not only to survive but also to regain their spirit to thrive.

As helping professionals, our work is guided by courageous engagement with those who have suffered traumatic losses and humanitarian crises. We cannot heal all the wounds, but we can create a safe haven where individuals, families, and community members are able to share deep pain and renewed strivings. Of value is our compassionate witnessing of their suffering and struggle and our admiration for their courage and endurance. When we shift focus from symptoms to strengths and potential, people find they have many unexpected competencies and resources and can build on them. We can rekindle their hopes and dreams for a better future and support their best efforts. We can encourage their mutual support and active strategies to overcome their challenges. Our response to tragedy can embody the humanity that binds us all together. We are, despite our differences, one human family.

CHAPTER 12

The Shared Human Experience of Loss

Professional and Personal Influences in Our Therapeutic Engagement

Grief can be the garden of compassion.
If you keep your heart open through everything,
your pain can become your greatest ally
in your life's search for love and wisdom.
—RUMI

All helping professionals are touched by death and loss in our lives and in our family legacies. These powerful experiences motivate some to dedicate their lives to careers in mental health, healthcare, pastoral care, or hospice services. Regardless of specialty, we will all see individuals, couples, and families facing heart-wrenching end-of-life or bereavement challenges. Sitting with clients who are dying or bereaved requires the clinician's emotional attunement, commitment, and nonabandonment. Some come to therapy years (or even a generation) later for emotional, behavioral, or relational problems that are entangled with earlier traumatic losses, often without noticing connections (see Chapter 10). Yet, focusing on such intensely painful experiences, like staring into the sun, can make us avert our gaze. We may avoid asking about significant losses, demur when clients seem uncomfortable, offer platitudes to cheer, or deflect to other topics. It requires us to approach death and loss issues without defensive armor and with openness, courage, and compassion.

THE THERAPIST'S RELATIONAL SELF
IN THE THERAPEUTIC ENGAGEMENT

The therapeutic relationship is at the heart of healing. Studies over decades have found it to be a common factor in effective therapy across models and specific intervention techniques (Sprenkle, Davis, & Lebow, 2009). As psychotherapy pioneer Carl Rogers (1961/2004) affirmed, it is the attitudes and feelings of the therapist, rather than theoretical orientation, which are most important. In systemic practice, the person, or self, is understood as relationally constructed through our most significant bonds, interactions, and experiences in social context, over time and across the generations.

Several founding family therapy developers, particularly Murray Bowen, Virginia Satir, and Carl Whitaker, considered it vital for therapists to understand the personal issues and concerns they bring to the therapeutic engagement. Even Salvador Minuchin, whose early structural model focused on skills and techniques, came to recognize that therapists themselves were the more important instrument of change. Believing we need to understand our own background to do this, he shared stories from his early life experience to make visible the values and experiences he brought to the therapeutic encounter (Minuchin, 1993).

For Harry Aponte (2022), the personal self of the therapist is an essential element in the therapeutic process because the human relationship with clients is the medium through which the work is done. The therapist's conscious, active, and purposeful use of self involves both empathic identification and differentiation of the clients' issues and concerns with those of the therapist. Aponte's training model emphasizes less therapists' self-resolution and more their capacity to engage in the therapeutic moment by gaining consciousness of their own related personal struggles and vulnerabilities. This enables them to resonate and empathize with the pains and issues of their clients. It promotes more intimate insight into what clients are experiencing and facilitates greater intuition into the dynamics of those experiences.

Aponte also incorporates a concern for the cultural and spiritual dimensions of peoples' functioning and the sociopolitical influences in therapists' and clients' lives, particularly those that marginalize people because of race, culture, and socioeconomic status. When working with clients across differences in social location, culture, or faith, therapists need to reach within ourselves to be able to empathically connect in the deep common humanity of our own personal lives, while expanding this connection to include clients' social context—all in affirming that each person matters.

Susan McDaniel, Jeri Hepworth, and William Doherty (1997) noted the lack of attention in the medical field to the personal illness experience of therapists working with patients and families challenged by chronic illness and disability. To understand more fully the relationship between the personal and the professional, they and their colleagues shared case illustrations revealing the relevance of their own illness experiences to their care for others, the way they interface with concerns of the patients and families they work with, and the use of these experiences to form a healing bond in therapy.

Common Challenges in Addressing Loss Issues: Turning Away/Turning Toward

We all grapple with our mortality and with significant losses in our lives and our family histories. In engaging with clients' distress, it's normal for clinicians' own strong emotions to be aroused around fundamental concerns in our common humanity. Reinforced by cultural norms, social discomfort, and behaviorally focused brief therapy models, clinicians risk ignoring or minimizing loss when they offer bright cheer or only prescribe medications to relieve symptoms. Additionally, when clinicians carry our personal or family experiences of loss into the therapeutic encounter, our own pain or anxieties may become entangled with those of our clients. In our discomfort, we risk avoiding our clients' suffering and struggles, compounding their pain, or abandoning them in their search for meaning and healing.

In gaining awareness and understanding of our contribution to the therapeutic encounter, we can more fully support our clients' process of grieving, meaning making, and coming to terms with death, dying, and loss. When a patient or client we have cared deeply about dies, we may be surprised by the intensity of our grief and may suppress it without acknowledgment and support. Working with the complicated grief of loved ones can be overwhelming, arousing our sense of helplessness and hopelessness: we are powerless to stop or reverse death. If our own painful or unattended loss experiences are reactivated, our distress is compounded. Being fully present with our patients and families may not sound like doing much, but it is the most important and difficult challenge in our therapeutic work.

Compassion Fatigue and Vicarious Resilience

The cumulative emotional strains from bearing witness to extreme suffering, powerlessness, and disruption often place helping professionals at risk for vicarious or secondary trauma and symptoms of burnout over time. Listening and responding empathically to intensely distressing accounts and ongoing struggles can affect helpers in compassion fatigue. Professionals who are isolated in their practice often lack opportunity for communication, understanding, and emotional support among colleagues. In large medical settings and community service agencies, the press of heavy workloads may not allow time and space for emotional processing of the death of a patient/client or the grief of their loved ones. Those working in oncology medical settings, palliative care, and hospice can suffer from the cumulative strains in caring for, and caring about, critically ill and dying patients and their families. It's vital to strengthen workplace resources for staff effectiveness, well-being, and resilience.

In collective loss experiences, such as natural disasters, mental health and healthcare professionals attend to survivors in acute distress while dealing with overwhelm and loss in their own lives. As therapists, we need to hold space for our clients' pain and support their healing process while making space for our own needs and those of our loved ones. For self-care, we need nourishing and revitalizing connections and respite from demands. Practicing relational resilience by engaging as allies with colleagues and building resource teams in our family, professional, and social networks, we can draw strength and inspiration from each other.

The concept of *vicarious resilience* (Hernandez et al., 2010) refers to the positive benefits for helping professionals when they expand the therapeutic focus to explore their clients' resilience in coping with and overcoming violent and traumatic experiences. Hernandez and her colleagues found that when therapists drew out people's stories of resourcefulness, such as remarkable courage, perseverance, and inventiveness, alongside accounts of their suffering and struggles, the therapists were deeply inspired and reinvigorated in their own work and personal lives, often in transformative ways. Most benefited from witnessing and reflecting on human beings' immense capacity to heal. They also learned from their clients the power of hope and commitment and the value of spiritual resources, a dimension they had not appreciated from their professional training but now included in their practice. In their work, they gained efficacy in the use of self in developing time, setting, and intervention boundaries and in building supportive community networks. Supporting Weingarten's (2004) work on witnessing violence, they reflected that, at their best, they were able to work from a position of compassion, awareness, knowledge, and effective action.

These effects generalized beyond therapists' work situation to significantly shape their perceptions of themselves, their relationships, and their environment. Their experience inspired them to reassess the significance of problems in their own lives, gaining tolerance for frustrations and an ability to adaptively reframe and cope with negative events. It also led them to clarify and strengthen their own values and perspectives on recovery and resilience. Working with multiple systems and witnessing transformations in clients' lives inspired some professionals to expand their work into teaching, writing, research, and activism.

Professional Constraints in Approaching Death and Loss

Professional training in the mental health field long recommended a therapeutic stance of neutrality to remain objective and unbiased with clients. Therapists were expected to be value free so as not to intrude into clients' beliefs or impose their own. Yet, clinical practice inescapably involves the interaction of therapists' and clients' value systems and constructions of norms, problems, and solutions. What we ask and pursue—or do not—influences the therapeutic relationship, course, and outcome. We best respect our clients by demonstrating active interest in the fullness of their experience in facing death, dying, and loss.

We can be blind to important issues in our clients' loss experience due to a confluence of constraints from our sociocultural, family, and professional norms and values. For instance, if we assume that matters concerning culture or spirituality don't belong in the clinical context, clients may sense our disinterest or discomfort and censor themselves from bringing these dimensions of their lives and loss into the therapeutic conversation. If we don't ask, they often don't mention them.

> Many years ago, a mother came for help with "communication problems" with two teenagers at home. It became clear that their immediate issues were related to the father's sudden death 4 years earlier (see Chapter 5). We worked together for several months, successfully addressing many ramifications of their painful loss and current relational strains. Long after completing therapy, I presented the (disguised) case for discussion in my clinical course on loss. A divinity dual-degree student in the class asked simply, "What happened to the family's spirituality with the father's death?" I was stunned. I had barely noted that the father had been a Protestant minister, beloved by their congregation. I replied honestly that I didn't know. I had never asked. And over the months of our therapy, no family member had ever mentioned faith implications, the father's role as spiritual leader, or the loss of their congregation.
>
> Further, the estranged eldest daughter, who had been closest to the father, was 17 at the time of his death. Taking flight from her painful loss, she had run off to live on a commune with a cult leader, severing all contact with her family and former life. The mother and I worked successfully over time to restore their contact. But we never explored the possible meaning and significance of the daughter's attachment to

the cult and its charismatic leader as their replacement for her father, the spiritual leader of her family and their congregation.

How had I not considered the spiritual dimension of loss in the family? At that time, in healthcare and mental health training, spirituality was regarded as not being the proper domain of clinical practice. Beyond noting clients' religious orientation, spiritual matters were to be left at the office door. While this has been changing in training and practice (Walsh, 2007), many therapists still feel ill equipped, hesitant to ask questions, and uncomfortable when spiritual concerns do arise—as they commonly do in facing death and loss. It's crucial to explore the significance of religion/spirituality in clients' experience, any spiritual concerns that contribute to suffering, and potential spiritual resources that could facilitate healing and resilience (see Chapter 3). When spiritual concerns are beyond the expertise of therapists, collaboration with pastoral professionals can be helpful to address both psychosocial and spiritual matters.

Personal Constraints: Exploring Our Own Beliefs and Experience

In recognizing spirituality as a significant dimension in human experience, therapists need to take stock of our own faith perspectives (including secular beliefs) and their influence in our therapeutic work. Surveys in the United States find that most therapists are less religious than most of their clients; many are unfamiliar with the faith orientation of those they work with. If our own religious experience is negative or devoid of spiritual meaning, it may constrain us from realizing the significant influence for others. If we and our clients have the same religious background, we must be cautious not to assume we share the same observance. If we view spirituality narrowly, as adherence to organized religion, we may not appreciate the varied ways people seek spiritual nourishment (see Chapter 3). Therapists and trainees benefit from deepening our knowledge of our family faith history and reflecting on our own spiritual paths (Walsh, 2009d). Such self-awareness increases comfort and openness in approaching the potential role of religion/spirituality in clients' distress and as resources for healing and growth.

As for many people, religion was a complicated matter in my multicultural family, with Catholic, Protestant, and Jewish roots, and rife with secret keeping, rejection, and painful losses. In early adulthood, I left it all behind, believing that religion was just not important in my life. Yet, that dismissal and my own unexamined spirituality contributed to my blindness to the spiritual issues in the previous family case. As I gained a deeper appreciation of my own spiritual complexities, it brought greater interest and comfort in exploring the spiritual matters in my clients' lives. Over time, like my parents, I've come to value a broad spirituality, with respect for the varied faith-based and nonreligious expressions of spirituality that can nourish and guide lives through adversity.

THERAPISTS' OWN EXPERIENCES AND LEGACIES OF LOSS

When attending to patients/clients who are struggling with death, dying, and loss, our own underlying pain, anxiety, or survival strategies, often out of awareness, leave us vulnerable to compassion fatigue and disconnection. In couples and families, with the varying impact and emotional intensity in relational systems, it's likely that some concerns may touch upon our own painful experience or anxiety about threatened loss. This requires our awareness of the interface issues in our therapeutic work. Yet, finding meaning in our own loss experiences can also enrich our practice.

Finding Light in the Shadow of Death

For family therapy educator Dorothy Becvar, the catalyst in exploring death and grief was the death of her 22-year-old son—the most devastating event of her life (Becvar, 2001). In her healing journey over many years, her search for explanations and understanding led to both a loss of fear of death and a much greater appreciation for life. It stoked her passion for helping people living in the shadow of death and increased her sensitivity to the dilemmas in this work.

As Becvar advised, from our own experience, professionals can find it deeply meaningful to help clients become more sensitive to the preciousness of life, the insight that change is the norm, that nothing stays the same, and we are always in transition. In helping them to reclaim their lives, these insights can also enhance our ability to savor sweet moments and contacts with others and to withstand periods of loss and despair, which are inevitable in our life passage.

Facing Our Mortality

I've come close to my own death—twice—jolting my awareness that life can end abruptly, at any moment, even when one is young and healthy. When I was in the Peace Corps in Morocco, enjoying a swim with a friend at a beach on the Atlantic coast, we both nearly drowned when we were swept out in a riptide and could not overcome the pull out to sea. Thankfully, we were rescued by two brave souls who risked their lives. But that terror has remained viscerally in my fear of drowning, even decades later. On a recent visit to the Dead Sea, stepping off a rock into deep water, I panicked, with arms flailing, despite "knowing" that the extremely buoyant saltwater keeps one afloat. My daughter had to carry me out, amid amused onlookers.

In my late 20s, I barely survived a head-on car crash on a two-lane country road on a sunny summer day in New England. An approaching driver passed another car on a curve, speeding toward me in my lane at 70 miles per hour. I suffered serious injuries, requiring several surgeries over the following months. It was a terrible time. I suffered flashbacks in traffic for many years, finally alleviated by eye-movement desensitization and reprocessing (EMDR). Yet, I also treasure memories of the caring support that got me through that ordeal: my dear friend and colleague Carol Anderson rallied to assure my best medical care; my Jungian therapist offered compassion and wisdom, and George Walsh read the entire Tolkien trilogy to me at my bedside.

THERAPISTS' OWN FAMILY EXPERIENCES OF LOSS

In the family therapy field, Murray Bowen, the first to attend to loss in family systems, once wrote about his own childhood experience: he grew up in a family of undertakers—which surely opened his consciousness to the profound impact of loss. I share here a few personal reflections from my own family experience and brief excerpts from writings by valued colleagues to inspire readers to explore your own legacies of loss and the interface with your therapeutic work.

Unspeakable Losses: My Family's Hidden Sorrows

In my late 20s, I was not prepared for my mother's death. Fitting the social expectations for young adulthood, I had left home and was pursuing my professional training and relational commitments. Like many peers, I had moved far from home. When my mother's health weakened at age 68, she was diagnosed with aplastic anemia and required regular blood transfusions. I shuttled back and forth across the country to spend a few days at a time and still not miss a beat in my demanding schedule. There was no personal leave allowed, without losing the entire training year. I felt torn: attending to the needs of families in my clinical setting while I wasn't supporting my own parents, a conflict that was intensified as an only child. My parents never complained, but my grandmother wrote to me, saying it was unconscionable for me to be caring for strangers but neglecting my own parents.

My mother's condition was fatal, but we never spoke of her dying, even as my parents made funeral plans. I kept thinking that she'd hold out longer. I had never faced the death of a loved one. When she went into a coma, I flew out and sat helplessly at her hospital bedside, too late to share our loving good-byes. The day after her funeral, I flew right back and hit the ground running at work, where I was praised for being so strong and responsible.

A few weeks later at dinner with my new in-laws, no one mentioned my mother's death. At the time, it was hurtful. Looking back, remembering how kind and loving Annie and Bernie always were, I'm sure they didn't know what to say without upsetting me, and they must have hoped that cooking a wonderful meal for me would help in my healing.

The American tendency to avoid facing the pain of death and loss, coupled with the image of the "rugged individual," perpetuates the faulty notion of resilience—just bounce back—be strong and put losses behind you. The expectation, from past developmental theory, that young adults have emotionally detached from their parents, contributed to minimize awareness of my loving bond with my mother and the significance of her loss. Only later did I begin to deal with her death, making time and space for grieving and reflection. I gained deeper comprehension that resilience involves a striving, over time, to make meaning and weave the fullness of the death and loss experience into the fabric of our personal and relational lives. In this way, my bond with my mother was not buried and lost, but transformed, deepened, and finding expression in my professional work and my personal connections.

Shortly before my mother's death, I pressed her to tell me about her young adult years, which she had never mentioned. I knew she had grown up in a French Canadian Catholic family. But the stories stopped there. She revealed that at 17 she had run off with her cousin Georgina to a convent, where they took their vows as Sisters of St Joseph, which pleased her devout mother (after her older brother Joe left the seminary to marry his sweetheart). Just months later, her beloved father, a railroad worker, was killed in a freak train accident in a blizzard. I hold precious today, my mother's only memento: the stone fob from the watch in his vest pocket, cracked down the middle when he was crushed between two cars of the train while trying to clear the tracks of snow.

During her convent years, my mother, a gifted pianist, was a highly admired music teacher, organist, and choir director. But her deep spirituality, humanity, and love of life were increasingly at odds with her hierarchical, ascetic, and cloistered life. With great anguish, she made the courageous decision to leave her religious vows for a "normal" secular life. In the 1930s, such a decision was rare, stigmatized, and raised questions of scandal. Her mother refused to see her and died of a stroke within the year. She was not told of her mother's death until after the funeral. The earlier loss of her father, the cutoff from her family, and the loss of reconciliation with her mother etched a deep sadness that my mother carried secretly all her life, a sorrow I could see in her eyes but had not comprehended.

After my mother's death, I was left to weave the hidden and disparate strands in her life together with my own experience of her. I reconnected with her relatives at a family reunion and gained a fuller understanding of her experience. Yet, mysteries remained, and I was left with regret over the lost opportunity to have important conversations through which I could know and love her better and answer questions about my own identity. I vowed to do it differently with my father while he was still alive. I stopped postponing efforts long intended to improve our relationship. But he was tough. I believed that the most dysfunctional families I worked with could change, but my father was hopeless. Fortunately, my efforts were encouraged by valuable coaching with Murray Bowen and by a cross-country drive with Monica, who wanted to meet my father—and liked him. Persisting in efforts to relate more genuinely, I wore down his resistance to revealing more about his life. I learned that he, too, had suffered many painful losses. I realized that despite the obvious differences between my parents (she was a gifted musician; he was tone deaf), they forged a close bond in making the most of their lives going forward—and an unspoken agreement not to ask each other about past sorrows.

My father's losses were of a different kind, beginning with hip dysplasia in infancy. With loving perseverance by his parents (and depleting their savings), he underwent three medical procedures in childhood, each time encased for months in a plaster cast. But each time, when the cast was removed, his hip slipped out of place again. My father lost his childhood, unable to walk or play with others, teased as a "cripple," and unable to start school until age 11, when his hip was finally repaired. Although bright, he was shy and gawky, and had a limp, with one leg noticeably shorter. The young children in his first-grade class cruelly taunted him until he dropped out, later completing education on his own. He then enrolled in a local college to become a pharmacist, working nights to pay his way. But the college closed, a casualty of the Great Depression. The pharmacist he worked for promised to leave him the business at retirement if he continued to work for little pay, but soon the business, too, was bankrupt. Again, my father's hopes and dreams were shattered. Yet, my parents, recently married, rebounded, moving to Kenosha, a small factory town, to forge a new path in life. They soon lost everything in a fire, when I was a toddler, and caring neighbors took us in until my parents were able to rebound. My dad's small business struggled financially over the years, despite his hard work. But they never gave up, eventually moving to California to start a new life when I was a teenager.

As a child, I had internalized the social stigma and shame my father experienced because of his disability, his social discomfort, and his struggles to earn a living. As I came to know him and learn of his life journey, my disappointment in him was transformed to admiration. I felt profound compassion for all he had suffered and gained deep respect and pride in him for the many challenges and losses he had overcome. As I came to see my father through new eyes, our relationship flourished.

At 74, my father was diagnosed with cancer and given only a few months to live. I was my dad's sole support, and I lived 2,000 miles away, with a 10-month-old baby and the responsibilities of a new associate deanship (see Chapter 4). Regretting and learning from my experience with my mother's death, I was determined to be there for my father. Yet, I now faced the dilemma I had noted in my research: the conflict of incompatible life-cycle imperatives: attention to my dying parent and my own grief juxtaposed with parenting priorities to meet my infant's needs. Our work can inform our personal lives: my research reinforced my sense of the vital importance of attending to my dying father and to my loss. Our pediatrician assured me that the baby's father and other caregivers could meet my infant's needs, but that I was the one who mattered to my father when he was dying. I mobilized resources at home and work and shuttled back and forth, to settle him temporarily in a partial-care residence, clear out his apartment, sort through his belongings and accounts, and handle funeral and burial arrangements—exhausting, with no relatives nearby, but supported by friends.

The last few weeks before my father's death were the most emotionally challenging for me. I found visits at his bedside increasingly awkward. Raised with cultural beliefs emphasizing mastery and control, I became a "doer," invested in goal-oriented action and problem solving. I found it difficult simply being with him in his dying. I kept wanting to leave the room to run errands for him. As I calmed my anxieties, I was better able simply to be present with him, keeping him company, stroking his arm, and holding his hand. I still have precious memories of those long days spent quietly together: at times laughing over *I Love Lucy* reruns on TV, at other times gazing peacefully out the window at the flowering mimosa tree as the sunlight streamed through it. Those last days, the hardest, were also the most precious time we ever shared. When my dad died, I grieved his loss, yet I was also at peace with our relationship. And I was grateful for the gift of love that, despite his own losses and life disappointments, he was able to give to me once I was able to reach out to him.

I was upset that my dad's brother did not fly out to be with him when he was dying, or come for the funeral. But I later understood that the sudden heart palpitations that made my Uncle Penny cancel his travel plans must have come from the ache in his heart at the impending loss of his only surviving sibling—and overwhelming memories of his other brother's death. In 1971, my Uncle Bob, a World War II war hero, had been shot in an inner-city robbery of their small business—and had bled out, dying in his brother's arms.

Recently, as I was reflecting on my family's many tragic losses, I asked my cousin Ken to share more with me about the impact of his father's death, since it was never talked about in our family. My Uncle Bob's murder tore through the heart of his immediate family, deeply affecting my Aunt Lottie and their daughter, Vicki, 22, and Ken, 24. It was an especially cruel death after all their father had endured in World War II combat. I learned that he had received a presidential award for leading his company across the Rhine River into Germany after surviving the consequential and deadly Battle of the Bulge.

At his murder, my aunt, who had just had surgery for breast cancer, was unable to function for many months in her grief. Vicki, away at college and near graduation, came home to live with her mother, taking on a devoted caregiving role for many years. She had a lonely life after her mother's death but found meaning in volunteer work in her religious congregation and in hospice services. Ken, recently returned from Army military service, tried to manage his grief to keep his new job and support his mother. They moved away to a quiet neighborhood. Yet they suffered heartache and financial strains for several years, consumed by legal proceedings that finally brought the assailant to conviction. Over time, that sense of justice and strong family bonds got them through.

I asked Ken what was hardest for him with his father's death. He said the most painful part was believing that his father might have survived the shooting if the ambulance could have reached him sooner—emergency medical technicians did not exist at that time. He paused to note his extreme pride when his son, Robert, named for his grandfather, became an EMT to save lives.

Ken said he was also troubled by the family's financial plight: they lost their sole source of income and incurred huge expenses in their lengthy legal efforts. There was no law at that time to compensate families bereaved by homicide. Ken was determined to do something so that no other family would suffer such financial hardship. Working as a technician for a local television station, he lobbied the top news bosses to urge passage of a new state law providing victim compensation. I told him how much I admired his efforts through such a terrible time. He said he had felt helpless—he couldn't bring back his dad, but here was something he could do. He knew his own family wouldn't benefit retroactively from the new law, but he knew his dad would be proud of him, and it helped him with his grief.

This is resilience. It's what you do with what you're given, when a tragic death cannot be undone. It's not surprising that I was drawn to my interest in resilience and my work with bereaved families throughout my career. A glance at my family tree across the generations reveals many untimely and traumatic losses. Yet, in learning more about those experiences, what has been most remarkable to me has been the ability of surviving loved ones to rise above tragedy to live good lives, to love each other well, and to do good for others.

Many years after my father's death, I opened a tattered old suitcase of his, which was still in my basement. I found awards and photos he had never mentioned in his modesty for his years of volunteer work for the Shrine Circus—supporting their hospitals for "crippled children" (as they were still called through the 1980s). I recalled his love of the circus and his comment, once, that he wished he could have become a clown to make children smile. Up to his final months of life, as coordinator of the Circus Daddies, he delighted in serving popcorn at the circus, making children smile.

It's not surprising that my parents were drawn to each other—out of their losses and, even more, in their resilient spirit. For the 20th anniversary of my mother's death, I wanted to find a meaningful way to commemorate her loss with my husband and daughter, who had never known her. Her gifts as a pianist and organist, and the love of music we shared, brought to my mind the carillon bells at Rockefeller Chapel on my campus at the University of Chicago. I called to ask if I might arrange a simple concert of bells on the evening of the anniversary. It was a cold December day in Chicago when we drove up and parked alongside the Chapel to hear the bells. The carillon musician approached us, inviting us to come in. She let us climb up to the top of the tower. As the bells pealed harmoniously into the crisp night air, we looked out at the starry sky and I felt my mother's spirit shining down.

It is never too late for rituals of remembrance that honor loved ones and foster connection. Recently, in remembrance of my mother's beloved father, I flew (with my dear friend Monica) to his hometown for the first time to visit his grave. I had planned this trip by first contacting the volunteers staffing the town's small historical museum. On arrival at the French Catholic cemetery, we found that all records had been destroyed long ago in a fire. And, sadly, the early graves were marked only by wooden plaques, with names no longer legible.

Practicing resilience, we went to see the museum volunteers. Anticipating our visit, they had accessed two newspaper notices of my grandfather's death in 1918, with details of the terrible train accident and his burial in the family plot—in another cemetery across the river. We dashed over, and I laid bright flowers on his grave and visited the adjacent grave of his mother, who also died young, my great-grandmother, Adeline.

Meaning making involves not only making sense of what has happened and all that was lost, but also finding meaning and purpose as we reorient our lives ahead. My life experiences, in facing the immediacy of mortality and in learning more about the lives and unspeakable losses in my family, brought greater clarity of vision (and less tolerance for bullshit). They sharpened my sense of priorities and catalyzed shifts in my life course, affirming deeper meaning, appreciation, and, above all, valuing our essential connectedness. I don't live in fear of dying and I am grateful for every day of life.

Uncovering My Family's Painful Experience of the Holocaust: A Journey of Meaning and Connection*

John Rolland, a leading expert on family challenges with illness, disability, and loss, recounted his experience of growing up with a deep sense that there were many untold tragic stories in his family (Rolland, 2004). His parents, German Jews, immigrated to the United States in 1935, barely escaping the growing atrocities toward Jews, but leaving behind their parents and other relatives.

> "My parents at times spoke in German. I didn't understand but it was clear that their stories were too painful. My father never spoke about his parents who died in a concentration camp, or of many other family members who perished. Once, when we went to see the movie *Judgment at Nuremberg*, my mother became so upset that we left. I never asked anything about that. It was clear that this was too excruciatingly painful."

When Rolland was in his psychiatry residency, his mother suffered a stroke and his first wife, Essie, diagnosed with a terminal form of cancer, underwent arduous treatments over the next 4 years until her death; his mother died shortly thereafter (Rolland, 2018). As both he and his father confronted the challenges of living in the face of loss, it was a turning point in their relationship.

---

*This section is based on Rolland (2004), a chapter in *Living Beyond Loss: Death in the Family* (2nd edition; Walsh & McGoldrick, 2004). Excerpted with permission of the author and editors.

"Shortly after, I visited his hometown in southern Germany, but didn't discuss it with him before I left. I took a walk to a hilltop castle over-looking the village—and later learned my father had walked on this path almost daily as a child. Then, in a strange and overwhelming experience in the Frankfurt train station, I started to cry, and I didn't know why. My father told me it was where he said his last good-bye to his family before leaving."

Rolland's family therapy training sparked him to do many hours of video interviews with his father, then 81, to uncover their family history. (He regretted not doing it earlier for his mother's stories and insights.) In his father's hometown, 299 of the 300 Jews were taken away to death camps. One elderly neighbor, Mrs. Altman, was left behind. Everyone perished in Riga, Latvia, where my grandparents were exterminated, except for one young woman, spared by a Nazi officer. Returning home, she conveyed the terrible losses to Mrs. Altman, who then wrote to my father. After the war, when he returned to Germany, Mrs. Altman gave him the few possessions she was able to preserve when the Nazis took everything from the Jewish homes. "A treasured silver Sabbath spice container that belonged to my grandparents has now come to me. As I was growing up, I didn't know what it was; it was just an odd object on a shelf. But there was such a huge story behind it."

"I was curious to learn about my parents' decision to leave Germany in 1935. Suddenly all restaurants had a sign, 'Jews are not allowed.' Jewish children were separated from gentiles at school, affecting my older brother's future. My father, a chemist, was not allowed to work. Fortunately, his education made it possible to immigrate to the U.S. I understood the strong value placed on education, as my father would say, 'It's the only thing that can't be taken away.' On arrival, as both a Jew and a German, he was advised to change his name, so he invented 'Rolland,' which would not be a giveaway."

In 1998, John was invited to Germany professionally, where he shared complicated feelings with his hosts, who had never spoken with a Jew whose parents had fled Germany. Several told of their very difficult relationships with their fathers as they questioned their role in atrocities. These collegial interactions were very meaningful. He then went for the first time to Wurzburg, his mother's hometown, where his parents met at university.

"There were stories about how my grandfather was falsely jailed and the family business, their home, and most possessions were confiscated.

That series of traumatic losses surely contributed to his early death of heart disease in 1938. My widowed grandmother, one of the last to get out in 1940, came to live with us until she died, when I was two, so I never got to know her.

"In planning my stay in Wurzburg, I chose a small rustic inn from a guidebook. When I got off the train it was raining heavily. I walked past other hotels, determined to reach the inn, although I knew nothing about it. On arrival, the inn was full. But the owner's family (not Jewish) kindly gave me one of their private rooms. Asked about my visit, I told them I came to see my mother's hometown. In hearing her name, they invited me to their dinner table, where the grandmother said, 'I knew your mother.'

"I didn't speak German, but using my high school French, I communicated through a French student staying at the inn. Another man at the table, a former city official, opened his wallet and took out a photo. He said he had been carrying it around for over 50 years, in case someday, someone would return for it. It was a picture of my grandparents' house, destroyed in an Allied fire bombing at the end of the war, when the Germans reversed their decision to surrender; over 5,000 persons perished in one night.

"The innkeepers took me to the site of the family home. When my parents went back for reparations in the 1950s, there was nothing left except the chimney and a rose trellis. I was powerfully affected when the grandmother said, 'This is your land.' In the yard stood one very old tree, all that had survived. The family then took me to the Jewish cemetery, where I found the graves of 40 relatives, and to the synagogue, now for the small community of Jews who returned.

"In my most powerful experience, they put me in touch with a local scholar and journalist (also not Jewish) who had written a book about the Jews of Wurzburg. He asked if I wanted the Gestapo files on my family. I was stunned; I had never imagined that possibility. He told me I had a right to the legal documents still on file and instructed me on how to get a copy. He warned that the officials would make it very difficult and, whatever they did, not to lose my temper. I went to the records office with my student translator. At first, they denied that my grandfather ever existed. After several hours (I just had to stay with it), a man finally entered holding the Gestapo files: my grandfather's picture was on the front with a large swastika underneath. He said they couldn't give them to me for a few days, knowing I had to leave that day. I saw a photocopy machine. I wanted to jump over the counter and either tear the files from him or send this man through a window. The French student gently put his hand on my arm, and I kept my temper, politely persisting until he gave in and handed me the files to copy. After returning home, I was unsure if my father would want to see them or if it would be too upsetting. He was very eager and translated them all for his children and grandchildren to have a record of the atrocities, documenting in bureaucratic detail the many arrests and harassments my grandfather had suffered. This record was very important in our family's healing process."

These experiences strongly influenced Rolland's personal value system and professional commitments. A year later, during the Serbian ethnic cleansing campaigns, he co-led design of family-centered programs for Bosnian and Kosovar refugees in Chicago. That led to developing a collaborative training program in Kosovo with local mental health professionals to assist families in recovering from the atrocities and losses in the war-torn region (Walsh, 2016c). He witnessed the bombing destruction and the personal suffering and endurance, hearing stories from Kosovar families that resonated with his own family's experience. "To be in a professional role to assist in their healing was also very healing for me, as was witnessing the resilience in families, as in my own family." Out of his experience, Rolland also reached a distinction: to condemn heinous acts by individuals or social/political systems without condemning an entire people and culture for all time. He notes:

> "Understandably, beneath my father's cheerfulness, there remained much deep pain and anger. But for me, through this process, I've come to see part of my life's work as fostering processes for reconciliation and healing, so we don't perpetuate a culture of retribution, an eye for an eye, which, as Gandhi recognized, 'only leaves us all blind.'"

Understanding Historical Legacies of Traumatic Loss in Ongoing Struggles for Racial Equity and Social Justice

Elaine Pinderhughes (2004), a pioneering clinical scholar with African American families, studied her own multigenerational family roots to better understand the historical influences in the ongoing struggles of Black families. As she experienced, clinicians' explorations of past traumatic losses in our families of origin can deepen understanding of our clients' experiences in historical and social contexts, broadening perspectives on their life challenges and on our own. Where there have been family secrets, hidden losses, and distorted communication, we may carry this aversion into our clinical work, not noticing or commenting on clients' painful losses, avoiding the heart of the matter and our own discomfort. When we also carry deep pain or fears from the past, we are more likely to turn away from understanding and addressing our client's most urgent issues, abandoning them in their quest for meaning and healing.

In training therapists, Pinderhughes shared her personal stories to illustrate the experience of millions of Blacks who have struggled to overcome the effects of lynching, riots, exploitation, and structural inequity for over 400 years. She offers examples from her own family's history to illustrate how multigenerational losses can affect persons struggling with ongoing threats to their lives and well-being. She describes how, in rural Louisiana in the early 1900s, her uncle, a physician, had given a white patient emergency treatment and was forced to flee with his family when warned that the Ku Klux Klan was on the way to lynch him. Her aunt (his wife) never recovered from the debilitating depression after that terrorizing incident. She talked longingly about the home and the life they left behind, and the catastrophic financial and emotional costs to the family.

Pinderhughes tells of her father, a highly successful dentist and a loving, though rigid, parent. When he was elderly, suffering from depression and dementia, one day he sadly and repeatedly mumbled, "It's a shame to kill a man without a coat." He was trying to say, "It's a shame to kill a man without a court." He was remembering terrorizing events in his childhood, when the Fourth of July was celebrated with the lynching of a Black man. After he fled from the South, he never mentioned this experience. Pinderhughes later learned of another hidden episode: "When my father returned South to introduce his bride, my mother, to his family, he was arrested in Alabama because it was assumed that his light-skinned wife was white."

In her genealogical research, Pinderhughes found records dating back to 1792 and her third great-grandmother, who was born a slave and later sold. Her family's sense of shame and pain about their ancestors' lives was obvious in their resistance to her work—and most of all in revealing the postslavery sexual exploitation of four female family members by Whites, including her mother and grandmother. Learning these secrets, however, and the pain about skin color preference helped Pinderhughes to understand her mother's depression and her abandonment in their relationship. (Her mother died when she was just 16.) "In my own family, energy tied up in maintaining related shame, pain, anxiety, family secrets, and communication blocks was freed up as pride replaced shame, clarity replaced confusion and ignorance, tranquility replaced anxiety, and connectedness replaced isolation" (Pinderhughes, 2004, p. 177).

As she experienced, the effects of being terrorized by ongoing traumatic circumstances not only mark the survivor in the moment but are transmitted into the future. These legacies are passed down to descendants through the compromised functioning of family members and, as well, by the ongoing lack of resources and active nonsupport of government and legal systems. She challenged those who think that focusing on the past only causes pain and reifies past victimization as a stance. She firmly believes that understanding the historical roots of ongoing inequities can humanize the struggle: therefore, she advocates moving from victim to survivor, striving to build better lives, appreciating the strengths of family members in the past and their coping methods to survive and adapt. In learning about transgenerational vulnerability, a client can better understand the roots of their parent's debilitating depression in the family's struggle for survival, gaining empathy for the parent's pain and strengths in making a life. Such work in therapy helps them to modify their sense of rootlessness and disconnection affecting their functioning. For Blacks, reconnecting with the past also reveals the vital role of religion and spirituality in providing a community and a belief system for transcending circumstances, as well as the power of music, from spirituals to gospel, jazz, and blues that express and transcend the pain and despair.

This expanded meaning making fosters transformation from an ongoing sense of vulnerability and powerlessness into a sense of power and determination to rise above past and present adversities. Still, Pinderhughes stresses that it is also essential to understand and address ongoing systemic patterns that perpetuate vulnerabilities and the changes required to end racial and other forms of discrimination and inequity that have life and death impact.

Systemic practitioners have become increasingly attentive to matters of social justice and view our responsibility as not limited to intrafamilial processes in the therapy room, but also in addressing larger system inequities and injustices. Toward this aim, David Denborough (2020), an influential community worker, teacher, and writer in Australia, recently took on a personal project, through the Dulwich Centre Foundation, to wrestle with the legacies of genocide. This project grew out of his commitment, as a white descendant of settler colonials, to engage with Australian history in ways that advance action toward decolonization and social justice. In his critical family history, a contextualized genealogy, he outlines the relationship of his family to Australia's Aboriginal peoples over time. He composed letters to his second great-grandfather and others who played influential roles in the colonization of Australia and the genocidal governmental policies that followed. Seeing meaning, emotion, and action as interconnected, he sought to honor the challenges and invitations from First Nations peoples "to bring our ancestors with us as we seek to work and walk together, and to try to be a good ancestor for future generations" (Denborough, 2020, p. 19).

OUR COMMON HUMANITY
IN THE THERAPEUTIC ENGAGEMENT

Today, robots are replacing human workers, and digital connections are replacing in-person interactions. Psychotherapy funding and reimbursement prioritize evidence-based, manualized treatment models, stepwise instruments, protocols, and online checklists, with intervention techniques presented as "tools in the toolbox." The role and person of the therapist have been eclipsed, despite decades of studies showing their importance.

If we check ourselves at the office door, we can't be fully present in our therapeutic engagement with clients struggling with painful end-of-life and bereavement concerns. As we've seen throughout this volume, each tragic death and loss, complicated by relational and situational factors, poses an array of common and unique challenges. Just as there is no single "healthy" way to grieve, or progression of stages of grief, or time limit on "normal" grief, our therapeutic work with the dying and the bereaved must be attuned to the many varied experiences, social locations, and cultural and spiritual orientations of our clients. In working with individuals, we need to attend to the reverberations of loss in their relational networks.

Grounded in systemic practice principles, the therapist's approach as compassionate witness and collaborator can itself be therapeutic, empowering clients whose life experiences are fraught with suffering and hardship. Because death and loss are universal challenges, their concerns may well touch upon our own vulnerabilities in our common humanity. Attention to our own experiences of loss and our family legacies of suffering, struggle, and resilience can be transformative in our therapeutic work and can enrich our personal lives and relationships.

Appendix

Suggested Resources and Readings

ONLINE AND HOTLINE RESOURCES

Centers for Disease Control and Prevention—Pregnancy and Infant Loss
www.cdc.gov/ncbddd/stillbirth/features/pregnancy-infant-loss.html

National SIDS and Infant Death Program Support Center
www.sids-id-psc.org

The Compassionate Friends—Supporting the Family after a Child Dies
www.compassionatefriends.org

National Alliance for Children's Grief
https://childrengrieve.org/find-support

Grandparents United
www.grandparentsunited.org

Compassion and Choices—Medical Aid in Dying
https://compassionandchoices.org/end-of-life-planning/learn/understanding-medical-aid-dying

Death with Dignity
www.deathwithdignity.org

National Domestic Violence Hotline
800-799-7233 (SAFE); *thehotline.org*

Centers for Disease Control and Prevention—Suicide Prevention
www.cdc.gov/suicide/prevention/index.html?CDC_AA_refVal=https%3A%2F%2Fwww.cdc.gov%2Fviolenceprevention%2Fsuicide%2Fprevention.html

National Suicide Prevention Lifeline
988 and 1-800-273-8255 (TALK)

Speaking of Suicide
www.speakingofsuicide.com/resources

Alliance of Hope for Suicide Loss Survivors
https://allianceofhope.org

International Suicide and Disaster Resources
Live Life: An Implementation Guide for Suicide Prevention in Countries. Geneva, Switzerland: World Health Organization, 2021 (available at *www.who.int/ publications/i/item/9789240026629*)

Disaster Resources for Children and Teens
www.childrenspsychologicalhealthcenter.org/resources/disaster-resources-for-children-teens

Podcast on Loss and Grief: *All There Is with Anderson Cooper*
www.cnn.com/audio/podcasts/all-there-is-with-anderson-cooper

BOOKS ON LOSS AND GRIEF

Elizabeth Alexander, *The Light of the World: A Memoir*
Julian Barnes, *Nothing to Be Frightened Of* and *Levels of Life*
Kate Bowler, *Everything Happens for a Reason: And Other Lies I've Loved*
Marion Coutts, *The Iceberg: A Memoir*
Joan Didion, *The Year of Magical Thinking*
Atul Gawande, *Being Mortal: Medicine and What Matters in the End*
Donald Hall, *The Best Day the Worst Day: Life with Jane Kenyon*
Kay Redfield Jamison, *Nothing Was the Same*
Paul Kalanithi, *When Breath Becomes Air*
Jon Katz, *Going Home: Finding Peace When Pets Die*
C. S. Lewis, *A Grief Observed*
Joyce Carol Oates, *A Widow's Story: A Memoir* and *Breathe: A Novel*
David Plante, *The Pure Lover: A Memoir of Grief*
Therese Rando, *How to Go on Living When Someone You Love Dies*
Anne Roiphe, *Epilogue: A Memoir*
Oliver Sacks, *Gratitude*
Kathryn Schulz, *Lost and Found*
Phyllis Silverman and Madelyn Kelley, *A Parents' Guide to Raising Grieving Children*
Karen Speerstra and Herbert Anderson, *The Divine Art of Dying: Living Well to Life's End*
Abigail Thomas, *A Three Dog Life*

References

Acosta, K. L. (2017). In the event of death: Lesbian families' plans to preserve step-parent–child relationships. *Family Relations, 66*(2), 244–257.

American Psychiatric Association. (2013). *Diagnostic and statistical manual of mental disorders* (5th ed.). Arlington, VA: Author.

American Psychiatric Association. (2022). *Diagnostic and statistical manual of mental disorders* (5th ed., text rev.). Arlington, VA: Author.

Anderson, H. (2009). Collaborative practice: Relationships and conversations that make a difference. In J. H. Bray & M. Stanton (Eds.), *The Wiley-Blackwell handbook of family psychology* (pp. 300–313). New York: Wiley-Blackwell.

Angelou, M. (2004). *The collected autobiographies of Maya Angelou.* New York: Modern Library Edition.

Antonovsky, A., & Sourani, T. (1988). Family sense of coherence and family adaptation. *Journal of Marriage and the Family, 50,* 79–92.

Aponte, H. J. (2022). The soul of therapy: The therapist's use of self in the therapeutic relationship. *Contemporary Family Therapy, 44,* 136–143.

Attig, T. (2011). *How we grieve: Relearning the world* (rev. ed.). New York: Oxford University Press.

Barboza, J., & Seedall, R. (2021, October 29). Evaluating the relationship between family resilience and grief-related symptoms: A preliminary analysis. *Death Studies,* 1–11. Online ahead of print.

Barboza, J., Seedall, R., & Neimeyer, R. A. (2022). Meaning co-construction: Facilitating shared family meaning-making in bereavement. *Family Process, 61*(1), 7–24.

Barrett, M. J., & Stone-Fish, L. (2014). *Treating complex trauma: A relational blueprint for collaboration and change.* New York: Routledge.

Bartel, B. T. (2020). Families grieving together: Integrating the loss of a child through ongoing relational connections. *Death Studies, 44*(8), 498–509

Bateson, G. (1979). *Mind and nature: A necessary unity.* New York: Dutton.

Becker, E. (1973). *The denial of death.* New York: Free Press.

Becker, C., Sargent, J., & Rolland, J. (2000). Kosovar Family Professional Educational Collaborative. *American Family Therapy Academy Newsletter, 80,* 26–30.

Becvar, D. S. (2001). *In the presence of grief: Helping family members resolve death, dying, and bereavement issues.* New York: Guilford Press.

Blow, C. (2020, October 14). My brother died and reminded me of these life lessons. Opinion. *The New York Times. www.nytimes.com/2020/10/14/opinion/brother-death-lessons.html?action=click&module=RelatedLinks&pgtype=Article*

Blow, C. (2022, January 23). Death changed my life. Opinion. *The New York Times. www.nytimes.com/2022/01/23/opinion/life-changes-death.html?smid=em-share*

Bonanno, G. A. (2004). Loss, trauma, and human resilience: Have we underestimated the human capacity to thrive after extremely aversive events? *American Psychologist, 59,* 20–28.

Boss, P. (1999). *Ambiguous loss.* Cambridge, MA: Harvard University Press.

Boss, P. (2017). Families of the missing: Psychosocial effect and therapeutic approaches. *International Review of the Red Cross, 99*(2), 519–534.

Bowen, M. (1978). *Family therapy in clinical practice.* New York: Aronson.

Bowlby, J. (1982). Attachment and loss: Retrospect and prospect. *American Journal of Orthopsychiatry, 52*(4), 664–678.

Bowler, K. (2018a). *Everything happens for a reason: And other lies I've loved.* New York: Random House.

Bowler, K. (2018b, January 26). What to say when you meet the angel of death at a party. Opinion. *The New York Times. www.nytimes.com/2018/01/26/opinion/sunday/cancer-what-to-say.html*

Breen, L. J., Szylit, R., Gilbert, K. R., Macpherson, C., Murphy, I., Nadeau, J. W., et al. (2019). Invitation to grief in the family context, *Death Studies, 43*(3), 173–182.

Brody, J. (2020, January 20). When life throws you curveballs, embrace the "new normal." *The New York Times. www.nytimes.com/2020/01/20/well/live/when-life-throws-you-curveballs-embrace-the-new-normal.html#:~:text=For%20patients%20with%20life-altering,of%20the%20here%20and%20now*

Byng-Hall, J. (2004). Loss and family scripts. In F. Walsh & M. McGoldrick (Eds.), *Living beyond loss: Death in the family* (pp. 85–98). New York: Norton.

Callimachi, R. (2021, July 19). Lost lives, lost culture: The forgotten history of indigenous boarding schools. *The New York Times. www.nytimes.com/2021/07/19/us/us-canada-indigenous-boarding-residential-schools.html?action=click&module=Top%20Stories&pgtype=Homepage*

Carr, D., & Jeffreys, J. F.(2010). Spousal bereavement in later life. In R. Neimeyer, D. Harris, H. Winokuer, & G. Thornton (Eds.), *Grief and bereavement in contemporary society: Bridging research and practice* (pp. 81–92). New York: Routledge.

Case, A., & Deaton, A. (2021, March 8). Life expectancy in adulthood is falling for those without a BA degree, but as educational gaps have widened, racial gaps have narrowed. *Proceedings of the National Academy of Sciences, 118*(11), e2024777118.

Caserta, M. S., Lund, D. A., Ulz, R. L., & Tabler, J. L. (2016). "One size does not fit all"—Partners in hospice care, an individualized approach to bereavement intervention. *OMEGA—Journal of Death and Dying, 73,* 107–125.

Catherall, D. R. (Ed.). (2004). *Handbook of stress, trauma, and the family.* New York: Brunner-Routledge.

Centers for Disease Control and Prevention. (2022a). Leading causes of death. *www.cdc.gov/nchs/fastats/leading-causes-of-death.htm*

Centers for Disease Control and Prevention. (2022b). Suicide rising across the U.S. *www.cdc.gov/suicide/facts*

Central Conference of American Rabbis. (1992). *Gates of prayer for weekdays and at a house of mourning: A gender-sensitive prayerbook*. New York: Author.

Charles, L. L. (2020). *International family therapy: A guide for multilateral systemic practice in mental health and psychosocial support*. New York: Routledge. *doi. org/10.4324/9780429354748*

Coelho, P. (2012). *Aleph*. New York: Vintage International.

Dalai Lama. (2002). *Advice on dying and living a better life* (J. Hopkins, Ed. & Trans). New York: Atria Books/Simon & Schuster.

Dalton, L., Rapa, E., Ziebland, S., Rochat, T., Kelly, B., Hanington, L., et al. (2019). Communication with children and adolescents about the life-threatening condition of their parent. *The Lancet, 393*(10176), 1164–1176.

DeFrain, J. (1991). Learning about grief from normal families: SIDS, stillbirth, and miscarriage. *Journal of Marital and Family Therapy, 17*, 215–232.

Deloria, V., Jr. (1994). *God is red: A native view of religion* (2nd ed.). Golden, CO: Fulcrum.

Denborough, D. (2012). *Collective narrative practice: Responding to individuals, groups, and communities who have experienced trauma*. Adelaide, Australia: Dulwich Centre Press.

Denborough, D. (2020). *Unsettling Australian histories: Letters to ancestry from a great-great grandson*. Adelaide, Australia: Dulwich Centre Foundation.

de Shazer, S. (1985). *Keys to solutions in brief therapy*. New York: Norton.

Didion, J. (2005). *The year of magical thinking*. New York: Vintage Books.

Doka, K. (2002). *Disenfranchised grief*. Champaign, IL: Research Press.

Emmerik, A., Kamphuis, A., Hulsbosch, P., & Emmelkamp, P. (2002). Single session debriefing after psychological trauma: A meta-analysis. *Lancet, 360*, 766–771.

Engel, G. (1961). Is grief a disease? A challenge for medical research. *Psychosomatic Medicine, 23*, 18–22.

Ennis, J., & Majid, U. (2021). "Death from a broken heart": A systematic review of the relationship between spousal bereavement and physical and physiological health outcomes. *Death Studies, 45*(7), 538–551.

Fadel, L., Jarenwattananon, P., & Hodges, L. (2021, September 1). His family fled Afghanistan 30 years ago. Now he's watching it happen again. All Things Considered. NPR. *www.npr.org/2021/09/01/1033374401/his-family-fled-afghanistan-30-years-ago-now-hes-watching-it-happen-again*

Falicov, C. (2014). *Latino families in therapy* (2nd ed.). New York: Guilford Press.

Falicov, C. J. (2016). The multiculturalism and diversity of families. In T. Sexton & J. Lebow (Eds.), *Handbook of family therapy* (pp. 66–85). New York: Routledge.

Fausset, R. (2019, June 13). How New Orleans celebrates its dead. *The New York Times. www.nytimes.com/interactive/2019/06/13/us/new-orleans-funerals.html?s*

Figley, C. (Ed.). (2002). *Treating compassion fatigue*. New York: Brunner-Routledge.

Fine, A., & Beck, A. (2019). Understanding our kinship with animals: Input for health care professionals interested in the human–animal bond. In A. Fine (Ed.), *Handbook on animal-assisted therapy* (5th ed., pp. 3–12). San Diego: Academic Press, Elsevier.

Fishbane, M. (2019). Healing intergenerational wounds. *Family Process, 58*(4), 796–818.

Flaskas, C. (2007). Holding hope and hopelessness: Therapeutic engagements with the balance of hope. *Journal of Family Therapy, 29*(2), 186–202.

Frankl, V. (2006). *Man's search for meaning.* New York: Beacon Press. (Original work published 1946)

Freud, S. (1957). Mourning and melancholia. In J. Strachey (Ed. & Trans.), *The standard edition of the complete works of Sigmund Freud* (Vol. 14, pp. 237–260). New York: Basic Books (Original work published 1917)

Gardiner, A. (2021, September 8). Wildfires took these families' homes. Here's why they stay. *The New York Times. www.nytimes.com/interactive/2021/09/07/us/oregon-wildfires.html*

Gawande, A. (2014). *Being mortal: Medicine and what matters in the end.* New York: Holt.

Gay, R. (Ed.). (2020). *The selected works of Audre Lorde.* New York: Norton.

Gil, E. (2014). Art therapy for processing children's traumatic grief and loss. In B. E. Thompson & R. Neimeyer (Eds.), *Grief and the expressive arts* (pp. 19–23). New York: Routledge.

Girwitz, A., Forgatch, M., & Wieling, E. (2008). Parenting practices as potential mechanisms for child adjustment following mass trauma. *Journal of Marital and Family Therapy, 34,* 177–192.

Gorman-Smith, D., Henry, D., & Tolan, P. (2004). Exposure to community violence and violence perpetration: The protective effects of family functioning. *Journal of Clinical Child and Adolescent Psychology, 33,* 439–449.

Greeff, A. P., & Human, B. (2004). Resilience in families in which a parent has died. *American Journal of Family Therapy, 32*(1), 27–42.

Greeff, A. P., & Joubert, A.-M. (2007). Spirituality and resilience in families in which a parent has died. *Psychological Reports, 100*(3), 897–900.

Greeff, A., Vansteenwegen, A., & Herbiest, T. (2011). Indicators of family resilience after the death of a child. *Omega, 63,* 343–358.

Griffin, B. J., Purcell, N., Burkman, K., Litz, B. T., Bryan, C. J., Schmitz, M., et al. (2019). Moral injury: An integrative review. *Journal of Traumatic Stress, 32*(3), 350–362.

Gruber, S. (2019, July 25). Living intimately with thoughts of death. *New York Times. www.nytimes.com/2019/07/25/well/live/living-intimately-with-thoughts-of-death.html*

Haas, A. P., Eliason, M., Mays, V. M., Mathy, R. M., Cochran, S. D., D'Augelli, A. R., et al. (2010). Suicide and suicide risk in lesbian, gay, bisexual, and transgender populations: Review and recommendations. *Journal of Homosexuality, 58,* 10–51.

Hardy, K. V. (2023). *Racial trauma: Clinical strategies and techniques for healing invisible wounds.* New York: Norton.

Hargrave, T., & Zasowski, N. (2016). *Families and forgiveness: Healing wounds in the intergenerational family* (2nd ed.). New York: Routledge.

Harris, D. (2020). *Non death loss and grief: Context and clinical implications.* New York: Routledge.

Harris, D., & Bordere, T. (Eds.). (2016). *Handbook of social justice in loss and grief: Diversity, equity, and inclusion.* New York: Routledge.

Harrison, T., & Connery, H. (2019). *The complete family guide to addiction.* New York: Guilford Press.

Hayslip, B., & Kaminski, P. (2005). Grandparents raising their grandchildren: A review of the literature and suggestions for practice. *The Gerontologist, 45,* 262–269.

Hedtke, L. (2012). *Bereavement support groups: Breathing life into stories of the dead.* Chagrin Falls, OH: Taos Institute.

Hemon, A. (2014). *The book of my lives*. New York: Picador.

Hernandez, P., Engstrom, D., & Gangsei, D. (2010). Exploring the impact of trauma on therapists: Vicarious resilience and related concepts in training. *Journal of Systemic Therapies, 29,* 67–83.

Hooghe, A., & Neimeyer, R. A. (2013). Family resilience in the wake of loss: A meaning-oriented contribution. In D. S. Becvar (Ed.), *Handbook of family resilience* (pp. 269–284). New York: Springer.

Hooghe, A., Rosenblatt, P., & Rober, P. (2017). "We hardly ever talk about it": Emotional attunement in couples after a child's death. *Family Process, 57*(1), 226–240.

Imber-Black, E. (Ed.). (1993). *Secrets in families and family therapy*. New York: Norton.

Imber-Black, E. (2012). The value of rituals in family life. In F. Walsh (Ed.), *Normal family processes* (4th ed., pp. 483–497). New York: Guilford Press.

Infurna, F. J., & Luthar, S. S. (2017). The multidimensional nature of resilience to spousal loss. *Journal of Personality and Social Psychology, 112*(6), 926–947.

International Medical Corps. (2017). Approach to Mental Health and Psychosocial Support (MHPSS). *https://cdn1.internationalmedicalcorps.org/wp-content/uploads/2017/07/International-Medical-Corps-2012-Our-Approach-to-Mental-Health-Psychosocial-Support.pdf*

Jamison, K. R. (1999). *Night falls fast: Understanding suicide*. New York: Knopf Borzoi Books.

Janoff-Bulman, R. (1992). *Shattered assumptions: Towards a new psychology of trauma*. New York: Free Press.

Johnson, S. (2019). *Attachment theory in practice: Emotionally focused therapy (EFT) with individuals, couples, and families*. New York: Guilford Press.

Jones, L. (2020). Grief and loss in displaced and refugee families. In S. Song & P. Ventevogel (Eds.), *Child, adolescent, and family refugee mental health: A global perspective* (pp. 123–149). New York: Springer.

Jordan, J., & McIntosh, J. L. (Eds.). (2011). *Grief after suicide: Understanding the consequences and caring for the survivors*. New York: Routledge.

Judd, A. (2022, August 31). The right to keep pain private. *The New York Times. www.nytimes.com/2022/08/31/opinion/ashley-judd-naomi-suicide.html*

Kalanithi, P. (2014, January 25). How long have I got left? Opinion. *The New York Times. www.nytimes.com/2014/01/25/opinion/sunday/how-long-have-i-got-left.html*

Kalanithi, P. (2016). *When breath becomes air*. New York: Random House.

Kaslow, N. J., Samples, T. S., Rhodes, M., & Gantt, S. (2011). A family-oriented and culturally sensitive postvention approach with suicide survivors. In J. Jordan & J. McIntosh (Eds.), *Grief after suicide* (pp. 301–323). New York: Routledge.

Killgore, W., Cloonan, S., Taylor, E., & Dailey, N. (2020). Loneliness: A signature mental health concern in the era of COVID-19. *Psychiatry Research, 290,* 113–117.

Killikelly, C., & Maercker, A. (2018, June 6). Prolonged grief disorder for ICD-11: The primacy of clinical utility and international applicability. *European Journal of Psychotraumatology, 8*(Suppl. 6), 1476441.

King, B. J. (2013). *How animals grieve*. Chicago: University of Chicago Press.

King, D. A., & Quill, T. (2006). Working with families in palliative care: One size does not fit all. *Journal of Palliative Medicine, 9*(3), 704–715.

King, D. A., & Wynne, L. C. (2004). The emergence of "family integrity" in later life. *Family Process, 43*(1), 7–21.

Kirmayer, L. J., Dandeneau, S., Marshall, E., Phillips, M. K., & Williamson, K. J. (2011). Rethinking resilience from indigenous perspectives. *Canadian Journal of Psychiatry, 56,* 84–91.

Kissane, D. W., Zaider, T. I., Li, Y., Hichenberg, S., Schuler, T., Lederberg, M., et al. (2016). Randomized controlled trial of family therapy in advanced cancer continued into bereavement. *Journal of Clinical Oncology, 34,* 1921–1927.

Klass, D., Silverman, P. R., & Nickman, S. (2014). *Continuing bonds: New understandings of grief.* New York: Taylor & Francis.

Kleinman, A. (2012). Culture, bereavement, and psychiatry. *The Lancet, 379*(9816), 608–609.

Kliman, G. (2007). Facilitating effective coping in children following disasters. *Journal of the American Psychoanalytic Association, 55*(1), 279–282.

Koch, C. (2020, June 1). What near-death experiences reveal about the brain. *Scientific American. www.scientificamerican.com/article/what-near-death-experiences-reveal-about-the-brain*

Koenig, H. (2012). Religion, spirituality, and health: The research and clinical implications. *ISRN Psychiatry,* Article ID 278730.

Kübler-Ross, E., & Kessler, D. (2005). *On grief and grieving.* New York: Scribner.

Landau, J. (2007). Enhancing resilience: Families and communities as agents for change. *Family Process, 46*(3), 351–365.

Landau, J., Mittal, M., & Wieling, E. (2008). Linking human systems: Strengthening individuals, families, and communities in the wake of mass trauma. *Journal of Marital and Family Therapy, 34,* 193–209.

Li, Y., Chan, W. C. H., & Marrable, T. (2023). "I never told my family I was grieving for my mom.": The not-disclosing-grief experiences of parentally bereaved adolescents and young adults in Chinese families. *Family Process.*

Lietz, C. (2011). Empathic action and family resilience: A narrative examination of the benefits of helping others. *Journal of Social Service Research, 37,* 254–265.

Litz, B., Liebowitz, L., Gray, M., & Nash, W. (2016). *Adaptive disclosure: A new treatment for military trauma, loss, and moral injury.* New York: Guilford Press.

Lorde, A. (2020). *The cancer journals.* New York: Penguin Books. (Original work published 1980)

MacDermid, S. W. (2010). Family risk and resilience in the context of war and terrorism. *Journal of Marriage and Family, 72,* 537–556.

Masten, A. S. (2019). Resilience from a developmental systems perspective. *World Psychiatry, 18*(1), 101–102.

Masten, A., & Motti-Stefanidi, F. (2020). Multisystemic resilience for children and youth in disaster: Reflections in the context of COVID-19. *Adversity and Resilience Science, 1*(2), 95–106. *https://link.springer.com/article/10.1007/s42844–020–00010-w*

Masten, A. S., & Narayan, A. J. (2012). Child development in the context of disaster, war and terrorism: Pathways of risk and resilience. *Annual Review of Psychology, 63,* 227–257.

McDaniel, S., Doherty, W., & Hepworth, J. (2013). *Medical family therapy and integrated care* (2nd ed.). Washington, DC: American Psychological Association Press.

McDaniel, S., Hepworth, J., & Doherty, W. (1997). *The shared experience of illness: Stories of patients, families, and their therapists.* New York: Basic Books.

McDowell, T., Knudson-Martin, C., & Bermudez, M. (2019). Third-order thinking in family therapy: Addressing social justice across family therapy practice. *Family Process, 58*(1), 9–22.

McGoldrick, M., Gerson, R., & Petry, S. (2020). *Genograms: Assessment and intervention* (4th ed.). New York: Norton.

McGoldrick, M., & Walsh, F. (1983). A systemic view of family history and loss. In M. Aronson & D. Wolberg (Eds.), *Group and family therapy 1983* (pp. 252–272). New York: Brunner/Mazel.

Mikulincer, M., & Shaver, P. (2008). An attachment perspective on bereavement. In M. Stroebe, R. Hansson, H. Schut, & W. Stroebe (Eds.), *Handbook of bereavement research: 21st-century perspectives* (pp. 87–112). Washington, DC: American Psychological Association.

Milman, E., Neimeyer, R. A., Fitzpatrick, M., MacKinnon, C. J., Muis, K. R., & Cohen, S. R. (2017). Prolonged grief symptomatology following violent loss: The mediating role of meaning. *European Journal of Psychotraumatology, 8*(Suppl. 6), 1503522.

Minuchin, S. (1993). *Family healing: Strategies for hope and understanding.* New York: Free Press.

Nadeau, J. (1997). *Families making sense of death.* Thousand Oaks, CA: Sage.

Nadeau, J. W. (2008). Meaning making in bereaved families: Assessment, intervention, and future research. In M. Stroebe, R. Hansson, H. Schut, & W. Stroebe (Eds.), *Handbook of bereavement research: 21st-century perspectives* (pp. 511–530). Washington, DC: American Psychological Association.

Neimeyer, R. A., Bottomley, J. S., & Bellet, B. W. (2018). Growing through grief: When loss is complicated. In K. J. Doka & A. Tucci (Eds.), *Transforming loss: Finding potential for growth* (pp. 95–111). Washington, DC: Hospice Foundation of America.

Neimeyer, R., Klass, D., & Dennis, M. (2014). A social constructionist account of grief: Loss and the narration of meaning. *Death Studies, 38*, 485–498.

Neimeyer, R. A., & Sands, D. C. (2011). Meaning reconstruction in bereavement: From principles to practice. In R. A. Neimeyer, D. L. H. Winokuer, D. Harris, & G. Thornton. (Eds.), *Grief and bereavement in contemporary society: Bridging research and practice* (pp. 9–22). New York: Routledge.

Nhat Hahn, T. (2002). *No death, no fear: Comforting wisdom for life.* New York: Penguin.

NIA Project, Emory University. (2021) Research and services to prevent domestic violence and support women who have been harmed. *https://psychiatry.emory.edu/niaproject*

Norris, F. H., & Alegria, M. (2005). Mental health care for ethnic minority individuals and communities in the aftermath of disasters and mass violence. *CNS Spectrums, 10*(2), 132–140.

Oates, J. C. (2021). *Breathe.* New York: HarperCollins.

Pargament, K. (2011). *Spiritually integrated psychotherapy: Understanding and addressing the sacred.* New York: Guilford Press.

Parkes, C. M. (2008). Bereavement following disasters. In M. Stroebe, R. Hansson, H. Schut, & W. Stroebe (Eds.), *Handbook of bereavement research: 21st-century perspectives* (pp. 463–484). Washington, DC: American Psychological Association.

Parkes, C. M. (2009). *Love and loss: The roots of grief and its complications.* New York: Routledge.

Parkes, C. M., Laungani, P., & Young, B. (Eds.). (2015). *Death and bereavement across cultures* (2nd ed.). New York: Routledge.

Paul, N., & Paul, B. (1986). *A marital puzzle*. Boston: Allyn & Bacon.

Perlman, L. A., Wortman, C. B., Feuer, C. A., Farber, C. H., & Rando, T. (2014). *Treating traumatic bereavement: A practitioner's guide*. New York: Guilford Press.

Pew Research Center, Religion and Public Life. (2015, May 12). America's changing religious landscape. *https://tinyurl.com/y953yrvf*

Pinderhughes, E. (2004). The multigenerational transmission of loss and trauma: The African-American experience. In F. Walsh & M. McGoldrick (Eds.), *Living beyond loss: Death in the family* (2nd ed., pp. 161–181). New York: Norton.

Prigerson, H. G., Kakarala, S., Gang, J., & Maciejewski, P. K. (2021). History and status of prolonged grief disorder as a psychiatric diagnosis. *Annual Review of Clinical Psychology, 17,* 109–126.

Prigerson, H. G., Shear, M. K., & Reynolds, C. F. (2022). Prolonged Grief Disorder Diagnostic Criteria—Helping those with maladaptive grief responses. *JAMA Psychiatry, 79*(4), 277–278.

Qin, A., Chien, A. C., & Dong, J. (2021, April 3). They survived Taiwan's train crash. Their loved ones did not. *The New York Times. www.nytimes.com/2021/04/03/world/asia/taiwan-train-crash.html?action=click&module=In%20Other%20News&pgtype=Homepage*

Rando, T. (Ed.). (1986). *Parental loss of a child*. Champaign, IL: Research Press.

Rando, T. (1993). *Treatment of complicated mourning*. Champaign, IL: Research Press.

Rogers, C. (1961/2004). *Becoming a person: A therapist's view of psychotherapy*. New York: Houghton Mifflin.

Rolland, J. (2004). Family legacies of the holocaust: My journey to recover the past. In F. Walsh & M. McGoldrick (Eds.), *Living beyond loss: Death in the family* (2nd ed., pp. 423–428). New York: Norton.

Rolland, J. (2018). *Helping couples and families navigate illness and disability*. New York: Guilford Press.

Rolland, J. S., Emanuel, L., & Torke, A. (2017). Applying a family systems lens to proxy decision making in clinical practice and research. *Family Systems and Health, 35*(1), 7–18.

Rosenblatt, P. C. (2013). Family grief in cross-cultural perspective. *Family Science, 4*(1), 12–19.

Rubin, S. S., Malkinson, R., & Witzum, E. (2012). *Working with the bereaved: Multiple lenses on loss and mourning*. New York: Routledge.

Sacks, O. (2015a). *Gratitude*. New York: Knopf.

Sacks, O. (2015b, February 19). My own life. Opinion. *The New York Times. www.nytimes.com/2015/02/19/opinion/oliver-sacks-on-learning-he-has-terminal-cancer.html?emc=eta1*

Saltzman, W. R. (2016). FOCUS Family Resilience Program: An innovative family intervention for trauma and loss. *Family Process, 55,* 647–659.

Sandler, I., Wolchik, S., Ayers, T., Tein, J.-Y., & Luecken, L. (2013). Family bereavement program (FBP) approach to promoting resilience following the death of a parent. *Family Science, 4,* 87–94.

Saul, J. (2013). *Collective trauma, collective healing: Promoting community healing in the aftermath of disaster*. New York: Springer.

Scheinkman, M., & Fishbane, M. (2004). The vulnerability cycle: Working with impasses in couple therapy. *Family Process, 43*(3), 279–299.

Senior, J. (2020, November 24). Happiness won't save you. *The New York Times. www. nytimes.com/2020/11/24/opinion/happiness-depression-suicide-psychology.html*

Shapiro, E. (1994). *Grief as a family process. A developmental approach to clinical practice.* New York: Guilford Press.

Shapiro, E. (2008). Recovery, of what? Relationships and environments promoting grief and growth. *Death Studies, 32*, 40–58.

Shear, M. K. (2015). Complicated grief. *New England Journal of Medicine, 372*, 153–160.

Shefsky, J. (2000). *A justice that heals.* Documentary film. Chicago: WTTW, Windows of the World Communications.

Shefsky, J. (2003). *Angels too soon.* Documentary film. Chicago: WTTW, Windows of the World Communications.

Smith-Stoner, M. (2007). End-of-life preferences for atheists. *Journal of Palliative Medicine, 10*(4), 923–928.

Sprenkle, D. H., Davis, S. D., & Lebow, J. L. (2009). *Common factors in couple and family therapy: The overlooked foundation for effective practice.* New York: Guilford Press.

Stinnett, N., & DeFrain, J. (1985). *Secrets of strong families.* Boston: Little, Brown.

Stroebe, M., & Schut, H. (2010). The dual process model of coping and bereavement: A decade on. *OMEGA—Journal of Death and Dying, 61*(4), 273–289.

Stroebe, M., & Schut, H. (2021). Bereavement in times of COVID-19: A review and theoretical framework. *OMEGA—Journal of Death and Dying, 82*(3), 500–522.

Stroebe, M., Schut, H., & Boerner, K. (2017). Cautioning health-care professionals. *OMEGA—Journal of Death and Dying, 74*(4), 455–473.

Stroebe, M., Schut, H., & Finkenauer, C. (2013). Parents coping with the death of their child: From individual to interpersonal to interactive perspectives. *Family Science, 4*(1), 28–36.

Stroebe, M., Schut, H., & van den Bout, J. (Eds.). (2013). *Complicated grief: Scientific foundations for health care professionals.* New York: Routledge.

Tedeschi, R. G., Shakespeare-Finch, J., Kanako, T., & Calhoun, L. (2018). *Posttraumatic growth: Theory, research, and applications.* New York: Routledge.

Thompson, B. E., & Neimeyer, R. A. (Eds.). (2014). *Grief and the expressive arts: Practices for creating meaning.* New York: Routledge.

Treadway, D. (2004). People die: Relationships don't: A reflection on surviving the suicide of someone you love. In F. Walsh & M. McGoldrick (Eds.), *Living beyond loss: Death in the family* (pp. 397–400). New York: Norton.

Treadway, D. (2022, July/August). Shattered by suicide: Helping families in the aftermath. *Psychotherapy Networker. www.psychotherapynetworker.org/magazine/article/2669/shattered-by-suicide/54afcf9f-a467-4d4f-90dc*

Ungar, M. (2020). Resilience and mental health: How multisystemic processes contribute to positive outcomes. *Lancet, 7*(5), 441–448.

van der Kolk, B. A. (2021). The body keeps the score: Memory and the evolving psychobiology of posttraumatic stress. In B. A. van der Kolk & A. C. McFarlane (Eds.), *Traumatic stress: The effects of overwhelming experience on mind, body, and society* (pp. 214–241). New York: Guilford Press.

Walsh, F. (1983). The timing of symptoms and critical events in the family life cycle.

In H. Liddle (Ed.), *Clinical implications of the family life cycle* (pp. 120–133). Rockville, MD: Aspen.

Walsh, F. (2002). Bouncing forward: Resilience in the aftermath of September 11, 2001. *Family Process, 41*(1), 34–36.

Walsh, F. (2003). Family resilience: A framework for clinical practice. *Family Process, 42*(1), 1–18.

Walsh, F. (2007). Traumatic loss and major disasters: Strengthening family and community resilience. *Family Process, 46*(2), 207–227.

Walsh, F. (2009a). Human–animal bonds I: The relational significance of companion animals. *Family Process, 48*(4) 462–480.

Walsh, F. (2009b). Human–animal bonds II: The role of pets in family systems and family therapy. *Family Process, 48*(4), 481–499.

Walsh, F. (2009c). Spiritual resources in adaptation to death and loss. In F. Walsh (Ed.), *Spiritual resources in family therapy* (2nd ed., pp. 81–102). New York: Guilford Press.

Walsh, F. (Ed.). (2009d). *Spiritual resources in family therapy.* New York: Guilford Press.

Walsh, F. (2010). Spiritual diversity: Multifaith perspectives in family therapy. *Family Process, 49,* 330–348.

Walsh, F. (2012). The "new normal": Diversity and complexity in 21st century families. In F. Walsh (Ed.), *Normal family processes: Diversity and complexity* (4th ed., pp. 4–27). New York: Guilford Press.

Walsh, F. (2016a). Applying a family resilience framework in training, practice, and research: Mastering the art of the possible. *Family Process, 55,* 616–632.

Walsh, F. (2016b). Family resilience: A developmental systems framework. *European Journal of Developmental Psychology, 13*(3), 1–12.

Walsh, F. (2016c). *Strengthening family resilience* (3rd ed.). New York: Guilford Press.

Walsh, F. (2019). Loss and bereavement in the family: A systemic framework for recovery and resilience. In B. Fiese (Ed.), *APA handbook of contemporary family psychology* (Vol. 1, pp. 649–663). Washington, DC: American Psychological Association Press.

Walsh, F. (2020). Loss and resilience in the time of Covid-19: Meaning-making, hope, and transcendence. *Family Process, 59*(3), 898–911.

Walsh, F. (2021). Family transitions: Challenges and resilience. In M. Dulcan (Ed.), *Textbook of child and adolescent psychiatry* (3rd ed., pp. 621–636).Washington, DC: American Psychiatric Association Press.

Walsh, F., & McGoldrick, M. (1988). Loss and the family life cycle. In C. Falicov (Ed.), *Family transitions: Continuity and change* (pp. 3–26). New York: Guilford Press.

Walsh, F., & McGoldrick, M. (Eds.). (1991). *Living beyond loss: Death in the family.* New York: Norton.

Walsh, F., & McGoldrick, M. (Eds.). (2004). *Living beyond loss: Death in the family* (2nd ed.). New York: Norton.

Walsh, F., & McGoldrick, M. (2013). Bereavement: A family life cycle perspective. *Family Science, 4,* 20–27.

Wang, L. (2019). *The farewell.* Film. Lulu Wang, Producer, Director. IMBd Studio.

Watson, M. F., Turner, W. L., & Hines, P. M. (2020). Black lives matter: We are in the same storm but not in the same boat. *Family Process, 59*(4), 1362–1373.

Webb, N. B. (Ed.). (2011). *Helping bereaved children: A handbook for practitioners* (3rd ed.). New York: Guilford Press.

Weine, S., Muzurovic, N., Kulauzovic, Y., Besic, S., Lezic, A., Mujagic, A., et al. (2004). Family consequences of refugee trauma. *Family Process, 43*(2), 147–160.

Weine, S. M., Raina, D., Zhubi, M., Delesi, M., Huseni, D., Feetham, S., et al. (2003). The TAFES multifamily group intervention for Kosovar refugees: A feasibility study. *Journal of Nervous and Mental Disease, 191*(2), 100–107.

Weingarten, K. (2004). Witnessing the effects of political violence in families: Mechanisms of intergenerational transmission of trauma and clinical interventions. *Journal of Marital and Family Therapy, 30*(1), 45–59.

Weingarten, K. (2010). Reasonable hope: Construct, clinical applications, and supports. *Family Process, 49,* 5–25.

Werner, A., & Moro, T. (2004). Unacknowledged and stigmatized losses. In F. Walsh & M. McGoldrick (Eds.), *Living beyond loss: Death in the family* (pp. 247–271). New York: Norton.

White, M. (1989). *Saying hullo again: The incorporation of the lost relationship in the resolution of grief. Selected Papers.* Adelaide, Australia: Dulwich Centre.

Whitney, C. (2016, August 4–7). *Strengthening resilience in refugee families impacted by trauma and loss.* Presidential Symposium: Providing Refugee Mental Health Services: Meeting Complex Needs, American Psychological Association Annual Convention, Denver, CO.

Winch, G. (2018, May 22). Why we need to take pet loss seriously. *Scientific American. www.scientificamerican.com/article/why-we-need-to-take-pet-loss-seriously*

Worden, J. W. (2018). *Grief counseling and grief therapy* (5th ed.). New York: Springer.

World Health Organization. (2019). *International classification of diseases and related health problems* (11th ed.). Geneva, Switzerland: Author.

Wortman, C., & Silver, R. (2001). The myths of coping with grief revisited. In M. S. Stroebe, R. O. Hansson, W. Stroebe, & H. Schut (Eds.), *Handbook of bereavement research: Consequences, coping, and care* (pp. 301–327). Washington, DC: American Psychological Association.

Wright, L. M., & Bell, J. M. (2021). *Illness beliefs: The heart of healing in families and individuals* (3rd ed.). Calgary, Canada: 4th Floor Press.

Yalom, I. (2009). *Staring at the sun: Overcoming the terror of death.* San Francisco: Jossey-Bass.

Index